TACKLING INSTITUTIONAL RACISM

Anti-racist policies and social work education and training

Laura Penketh

Dedication

For my mum and dad, Jean Taylor and Alan Penketh, who brought me up in an atmosphere of equality and social justice – values that I hope are reproduced in the following work.

First published in Great Britain in October 2000 by

The Policy Press
University of Bristol
34 Tyndall's Park Road
Bristol BS8 1PY
UK
Tel no +44 (0)117 954 6800
Fax no +44 (0)117 973 7308
E-mail tpp@bristol.ac.uk
http://www.policypress.org.uk

ISBN 1 86134 181 4

Laura Penketh is Lecturer in Social Policy at the University of Central Lancashire.

Cover design by Qube Design Associates, Bristol.
Front cover: Photograph kindly supplied by The Independent Syndication/ Andrew Buurman, 2000.
Printed in Great Britain by Hobbs the Printers Ltd, Southampton.

Contents

Acknowledgements

This book could not have been completed without the time, advice and support freely given by a number of people. First, I would like to extend my appreciation to all students and practice teachers who participated in the research, and to Chris Jones, who supported me throughout the research project. I am grateful to social policy colleagues at the University of Central Lancashire for their recognition of the pressures involved in writing a book while trying to cope with the increasing responsibilities and workloads faced by lecturers within academic institutions. My special thanks go to Alan Pratt – without his personal and professional support and understanding, the pressures would have been far greater. I am also aware of the pressures undertaking this project have had on my partner and my children.

Finally, I owe an enormous debt of gratitude to Michael Lavalette, who has proof read this work, and whose insights and observations have, as always, been invaluable.

Laura Penketh
January, 2000

A note on terminology

Debates regarding 'race' and 'racism' have become something of a linguistic minefield in recent years. For the 1960s' generation of activists, 'black was beautiful' and the struggle was for 'black power' – the term 'black' was used as a unifying concept drawing together all the victims of racism under one label. As the black activist Sivanandan stated, with regard to the postwar period:

> When we first came, racism was so undifferentiated, it didn't matter whether you were West Indian, African, Asian or Greek Cypriot. You were all the same as far as the system was concerned – if you were not True Blue or Dead White. (Sivanandan, 1991, p 35)

However, since the decline of the 1960s' social movements, of which the black movement was one, a politics of identity has grown which stresses the cultural difference and diversity of minority ethnic communities. Of course, there is a rich array of linguistic and cultural heritage among minority ethnic populations, which can have an impact on the social experiences of groups, but such approaches tend to emphasise 'difference' at the expense of what is common: the social and economic experiences of structural racism. It is also not the case that a rejection of the term 'black' is universal among people from a range of minority ethnic communities. For example, in the case of the Ricky Reel Family Campaign and the Michael Menson Family Campaign the label 'black' was positively accepted as part of the fight against racism.

In this book the use of the term 'black' is used to signify its role as a unifying concept in the struggle against racism. The debate regarding terminology, and the more recent development of the 'politics of difference', is explored further in Chapter One.

Introduction

The research which informed this book was carried out at a particular moment in the history of anti-discriminatory social work developments, when the Central Council for Education and Training in Social Work (CCETSW) incorporated anti-racist learning requirements in the Diploma in Social Work (Paper 30) (1989) (the professional social work qualification awarded after two years of education and training). This was an initiative which acknowledged the manifestation of racism in the social work arena, and made it a compulsory requirement that issues of 'race' and racism should be addressed in all aspects of social work education and training. These were radical developments which signalled a serious commitment by a state welfare organisation to tackle racism. For the first time, while they were undertaking training in social work agencies, students and their practice teachers (work-based supervisors) were given the responsibility for implementing anti-racist learning requirements.

The research project, which was instigated by the Department of Social Work at the University of Central Lancashire, initially set out to explore how far CCETSW's anti-racist learning requirements were achieved, and what barriers, if any, there were to implementation. It sought, through detailed information from students themselves, to identify as clearly as possible, any difficulties associated with dissemination and anti-discriminatory practice which they experienced while on placement in social work agencies. Interviews were carried out with a sample of black and white students in order to facilitate a comparative analysis to explore if there were similarities in experiences, or if 'race' and racism were more dominant factors in determining the experiences of black students. As practice teachers (qualified social workers within agencies) are responsible for supervising students, they too were interviewed to assess the impact they had on the placement experiences of students. In this respect, the research was concerned with contributing to a deeper understanding of racial exclusion and discrimination within the personal social services, at a time when anti-racism was becoming a fundamental part of CCETSW's legislation regarding social work education and training.

Interviews were undertaken with first and second year students and their respective practice teachers. In-depth semi-structured taped interviews were carried out with 20 students in a variety of social work settings. Each student was interviewed three times during the first year of the research project (1991) and half of the group were then interviewed again during the second year of the project (1992). Interviews lasted about two hours, and the length and number of interviews carried out facilitated a thorough and detailed exploration of students' experiences, and a chance to assess how experiences and perspectives developed and changed as placements progressed. The high level of contact with students was also constructive in creating an environment of trust and confidence, which made discussing issues around 'race' and racism less threatening. Practice teachers were also interviewed once during each student's placement, and again interviews lasted about two hours.

In the interviews, general aspects of education and training were explored alongside specific lines of questioning regarding black staff and client representation, the accessibility of anti-discriminatory policies, and the ability to implement anti-racist learning requirements. For example, students were asked, 'Do you have any black clients?', 'Are there sufficient resources to ensure effective service delivery for black clients?', 'Have you been informed of anti-discriminatory policies?', 'Would you feel confident in dealing with racism?', 'Have you experienced any form of discrimination?', 'Has anti-racist practice been on the learning agenda?'. Practice teachers were asked questions regarding their social work background, the time and resources available to supervise students, their feelings regarding the learning needs of black students and if they referred to or implemented anti-discriminatory policies.

As the first round of interviews were finishing, CCETSW's anti-racist initiative was coming under increasing attack by politicians, the media and sections of the social work profession, with CCETSW being accused of promoting a 'politically correct' policy initiative. Thus, at the same time as initial research interviews were beginning to reveal that institutional racism was fundamental to the experiences of black students, it was being increasingly problematised, criticised and dismissed politically and professionally. Over the next few months, as a result of the persistent political and media onslaught, CCETSW began to significantly retreat from their initial anti-racist initiative. This then opened up another series of questions. Why had there been such a backlash? Was the racism exaggerated? Did CCETSW's anti-racist initiative conflict with traditional social work practices? As a result, the initial research developed to look at a 'complete policy process', the routes and pressures promoting anti-racism, the experience of implementing anti-racist practice and the backlash against the policy.

More recently, the question of institutional racism and the way it blights the lives of Britain's black population has been brought sharply into focus by the murder of Stephen Lawrence and the inquiry into his death. The Macpherson Report (1999), like CCETSW previously, pointed to the damaging impact of institutional racism on policies, procedures and practices, and, like CCETSW, it too experienced a backlash, its recommendations being condemned by sections of the media, politicians and the Metropolitan Police. For social policy academics and practitioners who have to face up to the reality of institutional racism in Britain, CCETSW's experience from the late 1980s into the 1990s provides a fruitful case study and valuable lessons, as well as identifying areas of potential conflict. As the debate regarding institutional racism continues, the research on which this book is based remains timely and relevant for all concerned with tackling racism within a range of welfare institutions (see Denney, 1991; Gordon, 1992; *The Guardian*, 2000).

The CCETSW experience is in many ways being repeated in the 'post-Macpherson' experience. Given this, it is useful to ask a range of questions about racism and anti-racist practice of welfare activists and practitioners. Is it useful to describe Britain as institutionally racist? How can we implement anti-racist practice within welfare institutions? What is the range of barriers facing anti-racist activists? What lessons can we take from the CCETSW experience?

This book will begin to address some of these questions, opening up a debate within social work and social policy, both in the academy and in the field, over how we can deal with issues of oppression and discrimination within welfare organisations. Given this aim, the book is organised as follows: Chapter One analyses the concepts of 'race', racism and anti-racist practice, the development of 'race-related' legislation, and the assumptions underpinning each of these. CCETSW was heavily criticised for describing Britain as an institutionally racist society. Melanie Phillips in *The Observer* (1 August 1993) condemned social work training for expecting students to acknowledge "individual and institutional racism and ways to combat both through anti-racist practice", and to be aware of the "processes of structural oppression". This chapter sets out to defend CCETSW's claims and argues that social workers and social work education need to be aware of the reality and effects of racism in modern Britain.

Chapter Two moves on to assess the development of social work as a state profession. Categorisations emerged as analysis of interviews with students and practice teachers progressed. They reflect three general approaches by practice teachers to the role of social work in society, particularly in relation to social work intervention with deprived and marginalised groups, and their perceptions regarding the role of anti-racist perspectives in social work education and training. In doing so, the role of social work in society is explored, and views of poverty, disadvantage and inequality among its client groups. The tension between the caring and controlling aspects of social work provision is examined, along with the differing perspectives of social workers regarding their professional role. In doing so, three general categories of social worker are identified – 'conservative', 'social democratic' and 'radical'. How each of these categories perceives the nature of social work education, training and practice is explored. Defining social workers in this way is an heuristic device, but it points to something fundamentally important: not all social workers share the same values or the same conception of their role and function. 'Conservative' workers are more inclined to develop pathologising and controlling forms of practice; 'radical' workers view themselves as standing with clients in the face of a range of oppressions; the majority reflect a series of 'social democratic' assumptions about equality, justice and the possibility of welfare activity to improve gradually the lives of the very poorest in modern society. These groups differ in the degree to which they recognise the relevance of anti-oppressive theory and practice. On the basis of research findings, I suggest that radical workers are open to these developments, conservative workers are hostile, whereas the majority are unsure and non-committal. However, this majority, with appropriate resources and training, could have been won to anti-racist practice, but in an era of resource cuts, and an atmosphere of backlash, anti-racism has been seen as just another managerial requirement, another 'straw bending the camel's back to near breaking point'. Consequently, these workers appear to be a vital lost resource in the campaign to reinforce anti-racist practice.

Chapter Three explores the particular context within which CCETSW's anti-racist strategy developed. The late 1980s was not a period of significant 'Left advance'. Margaret Thatcher was enjoying her third term in office, and significant sections of the trade union movement (eg the miners) and municipal Left (eg the GLC, Sheffield and Liverpool Councils) had been confronted and defeated. Nevertheless, during this period CCETSW developed a radical agenda for trainee social workers that stressed class inequality and the structural and institutional nature of a range of oppressions. Why? Where did these ideas come from? These issues are addressed in this chapter.

Chapters Four, Five and Six present the research findings of a series of interviews held with students and practice teachers during the first two years of the new Diploma in Social Work course. They reveal the experiences of students, the difficulties the students faced within social work agencies, and the problems that practice teachers had facilitating anti-racist practice. Together they highlight some of the difficulties facing individuals (both committed and hostile) trying to implement anti-racist procedures within institutionally racist agencies.

Finally, Chapter Seven looks at the backlash against CCETSW and the focus placed on 'political correctness' (PC), an increasingly wide catch-all phrase utilised to attack any attempts to tackle social injustice. But again, did the linguistic emphasis of PC in any way prepare the ground for the backlash? And what was the interconnection between PC and CCETSW's programme? While defending attempts to control 'hate language', drawing on the works of Molyneux (1993) and Holborow (1999), I suggest that the main thrust of PC, like CCETSW's anti-racist programme, was to impose particular language and practice codes onto people, and it was this 'top-down' imposition that left it vulnerable and open to ridicule and retreat.

In the concluding chapter I return to the present and the continuing problem of institutional and structural racism in Britain. I suggest that the CCETSW experience provides some important lessons for those who wish to fight racism and to teach anti-racist practice to a range of welfare workers. In this sense it remains an important, and not merely an historical, piece of social policy development.

ONE

'Race' and racism in modern Britain

Racism continues to blight the lives of the black population in Britain today. It operates in the systematic discrimination which black people face in the labour market, and the housing, education and health services (Solomos and Back, 1996). It is present in the harassment that black people face at the hands of the police and the immigration authorities (Callinicos, 1993), as is evidenced in the fact that black people are more likely to be 'stopped and searched', arrested, imprisoned, and even to die in custody than whites, and are likely to be seen as perpetrators of crime even when they are victims (Bowling, 1999; Younge, 2000a). It also rears its ugliest head in the violence perpetuated against black people by racist thugs, shown most graphically in the murders of Stephen Lawrence and Michael Menson, but present on street corners, and in the violence against properties and homes across the country. As CCETSW noted, at the beginning of the 21st century racism within Britain is 'endemic'.

Institutional racism affects the representation and treatment of black people within a range of state institutions. For example, the 1997/98 Labour Force Survey revealed that:

> Unemployment rates were 6% for whites, 8% for Indians, 19% amongst the black community and 21% amongst Bangladeshis and Pakistanis [and that].... More than 40% of 16 to 17 year olds from ethnic-minority groups were unemployed compared to 18% of their white peers. (*The Guardian*, 21 February, 2000, p 13)

For those members of the black communities in work, their earnings are likely to be lower than white people in equivalent jobs. The Institute for Social and Economic Research found that between 1985 and 1995:

> On average, Pakistani and Bangladeshi men earned just over half the salary of their white peers. (*The Guardian*, 21 February, 2000, p 13)

Black people are more likely to live in inferior housing in run–down areas (Ginsburg, 1992; Law, 1998), experience higher mortality and morbidity rates (Skellington and Morris, 1992; Blackburn Borough Council, 1996), differential health provision (Skellington and Morris, 1992; Ahmad and Atkin, 1996), and are often subject to differential treatment in terms of educational provision (Troyna and Hatcher, 1992; Gore, 1998). For example, in 1999 the Children's Society revealed that black children are six times more likely to be expelled from school than white children (*The Guardian*, 21 February, 2000). These statistics were reinforced in the Macpherson Report that published the findings of the Stephen Lawrence Inquiry. Housing departments were seen to be too slow and bureaucratic in response to racist tenants, and in schools there was disturbing evidence of widespread racist attitudes among very young children, and a failure to implement anti-racist policies (*The Guardian*, 25 February, 1999). While *Statewatch* noted that within the criminal justice system:

> Black people are between four and seven times more likely to be sentenced to prison terms, and nearly eight times more likely to be stopped and searched by the police. (*The Guardian*, 21 February, 2000, p 7)

During the past decade the extent and nature of racism in British society has been given an increasingly high public and political profile, and the interpretation of racism has moved from one based on personal prejudice, towards an acknowledgement of its institutional manifestation. A major impetus to this debate was the murder of Stephen Lawrence in 1993, and the endeavours of his parents, Neville and Doreen Lawrence, to expose the racism of the Metropolitan Police in dealing with his death. In early 1997, a coroner's jury, after just 30 minutes of deliberation, returned a verdict of unlawful killing "in a completely unprovoked racist attack by five white youths" (*The Guardian*, 14 February, 1997), and in July 1997, the Home Secretary Jack Straw set up a judicial public inquiry into the case to be chaired by Sir William Macpherson.

The findings of the Macpherson Report were revealed in February 1999, and concluded that racism exists within all organisations and institutions, and is:

> ... deeply ingrained. Radical thinking and sustained action are needed in order to tackle it head on ... in all organisations and in particular in the fields of education and family life. (*The Guardian*, 25 February, 1999)

During the Inquiry Michael Mansfield, QC, acting on behalf of the Lawrence family, stated that:

> The magnitude of the failure in this case ... cannot be explained by mere incompetence or a lack of direction by senior officers or a lack of execution and application by junior officers, nor by woeful under-resourcing. So much was missed by so many that deeper causes and forces must be considered. We suggest that these forces relate to two main propositions. The first is that the victim was black and racism, both conscious and unconscious, permeated the investigation. Secondly, the fact is that the perpetrators were white and were expecting some form of protection. (Norton-Taylor, 1999, pp 22-3)

Mansfield went on to describe the racism which the Lawrence family had faced as they fought for justice, which included having their tyres slashed and their home being watched by 'threatening' white youths.

The conclusions of the Macpherson Report, that racism was institutionalised within British society, were a radical departure from recommendations enshrined in the Scarman Report (1982), the last major investigation into police racism in Britain, commissioned after the Brixton riots of 1981. Scarman had concluded that:

> The direction and policies of the Metropolitan Police are not racist. [I] totally and unequivocally reject the attack made upon the integrity and impartiality of the senior direction of the force. (para 4.62, cited in Barker and Beezer, 1983, p 110)

Evidence of the brutality of racist violence and how deeply entrenched institutional racism is has been emphasised since the murder of Stephen Lawrence in the deaths of Ricky Reel, Michael Menson, Christopher Alder (who died in police custody), and, more recently, 'Erroll' and Jason McGowan. It is clear that institutional racism is deeply embedded in the criminal justice system, but as various other studies show (see for example Lavalette et al, 1998), and the Macpherson Report emphasises, racism operates in all organisations and institutions in society, and blights the lives of Britain's black population.

The Macpherson Report was not the first time that institutional racism had been acknowledged by a state official or institution. Several years before the murder of Stephen Lawrence, the issue of institutional racism was being addressed seriously by CCETSW. This arose as a result of professional concern within the social work arena regarding the manifestation of racism in all aspects of social work education, training and practice, and led to a concerted attempt to develop a more radical anti-racist approach. There was increasing recognition and concern that the black population were under-represented, both as workers and as clients in social work agencies (Cheetham, 1987), and that when they were represented, they were often pathologised using negative and damaging assumptions, endorsing the superiority of white culture over others (Husband, 1991).

The direction taken by CCETSW came about from discussions that took place among both black and white sections of the social work academy and profession during the 1980s, in workshops, conferences and publications. As a result of these pressures and activities, in 1989 CCETSW introduced the *Rules and Regulations for the Diploma in Social Work* (Paper 30), which made it a compulsory requirement for students undertaking social work training to address issues of 'race' and racism, and to demonstrate competence in anti-racist practice. As a consequence, university courses and social work agencies were required to facilitate anti-racist training for students with the aim that, eventually, social workers in the field would be conscious of the nature of structural and institutional racism in British society, and would be able to support clients faced with such oppression.

In many ways this was a remarkable initiative, which represented a significant and important step forward. It emanated from a government agency and contained within its remit a recognition that Britain was an institutionally racist country, and that social work education and training should, as a consequence, be structured by anti-racist concerns and principles.

However, its successful implementation was impaired by a political, and in some cases, professional backlash, which denied the structural and institutional nature of racism, and accused CCETSW of being taken over by groups of obsessed zealots whose major concern was to express rigid PC values (Jones, 1993). Professor Robert Pinker, a prominent academic in the area of social work and social policy, expressed his condemnation of CCETSW's anti-racist developments, and his views reflect criticisms being articulated in other quarters. He stated "It was clear to some of us in the academic community that radical political elements had taken over the whole of the council's planning process" and that "there would be no avenues of escape for either staff or students from this nightmare world of censorship and brainwashing". He accused those involved in developing CCETSW's initiatives of believing that "oppression and discrimination are everywhere to be found in British society, even when they seemed to be 'invisible'" (Pinker, 1999 pp, 18-19).

The irony is that in 1993, the year of Stephen Lawrence's murder, while CCETSW was making a valiant and committed effort to challenge the institutional manifestation of racism within a state organisation, it increasingly found itself under attack by Right-wing politicians, sections of the social work profession, and the media, who denied their assertion of the institutional nature of racism within Britain, and ridiculed their anti-racist initiatives. It is perhaps no surprise that more recently, the Macpherson Report has experienced a similar response from the Metropolitan Police, Right-wing politicians and media commentators.

CCETSW's Paper 30 and the Macpherson Report are both a 'break with the past' in their conclusions that state institutions must move beyond analyses of racism based on personal and cultural prejudice, and that racism is much more than the sum total of the actions of prejudiced individuals. Instead, they focus on the need to recognise and challenge the structural and institutional nature of racism in contemporary British society. But what do they mean by this? What is 'race' and racism? Specifically, what is meant by institutional racism and structural racism? Answering these questions became a central concern for social work academics preparing Paper 30, but a rejection of their claims became central to the backlash against CCETSW. In order to assess the validity of CCETSW's case, therefore, it is necessary to review the ground on which the debate flourished.

The origins of racism

Racism is a relatively modern phenomenon that grew up with the development and expansion of capitalism as a global social and economic system (Miles, 1982; Fryer, 1984; Callinicos, 1993). It developed in the 17th and 18th centuries in order to justify the systematic use of African slave labour in the great plantations of the New World, when, during the 18th century alone, some twelve million African captives were transported to work on the plantations of North America and the West Indies (Blackburn, 1997). Slavery was not invented during the 17th and 18th centuries; rather it had existed in small pockets in different parts of Europe and the Middle East during the middle-ages. But:

> The slavery that did exist was not associated with black people more than any other group. Whites could be galley slaves and the word slave is derived from 'Slav'. (Harman, 1999, pp 249-50)

Patrick Manning has estimated that "In 1500, Africans or persons of African descent, were a clear minority of the world's slave population; but by 1700, the majority" (Manning, 1990, p 30).

The development of slavery escalated dramatically in the 17th century when Portugal, Holland, England and France began the commercial cultivation of tobacco and sugar in their West Indian colonies. At first the plantation owners met their labour demands by utilising the un-free labour of indentured white workers. Blackburn suggests that in the sugar plantations of Barbados in 1638 there were 2,000 indentured servants compared with 200 African slaves (Blackburn, 1997, p 230). But indentured slavery from Europe could not fulfil the labour demand emanating from the plantations and the owners increasingly turned to African slaves. By 1653 Blackburn estimates that the number of slaves in Barbados had risen to 20,000, while indentured servants numbered 8,000 (Blackburn, 1997, p 231).

Indentured servants and slaves worked, lived and rebelled together, and it was in response to these events, Blackburn argues, that the landowners and the political representatives sought to demarcate and strengthen the barriers between white servants and black slaves. Racism evolved therefore as a byproduct of the 17th-century slave trade. It developed to justify slavery, the barbaric treatment of black slaves and the domination of the world by Western Imperialism (Miles, 1982; Fryer, 1984; Ramdin, 1987; Callinicos, 1993).

Racism was based on the view that humankind was divided into 'races' reflected in distinct biological characteristics, with white 'races' being superior to black 'races'. Racial differences were therefore socially constructed, and created as part of an historically specific relationship of oppression (Callinicos, 1993). These racist ideologies constructed, promoted and disseminated images of black populations as, for example, savage, unintelligent, dirty, and licentious (Fryer, 1984). Edward Long (the son of a Jamaican planter) wrote in his *Universal history* (1736-65) that Africans were:

> ... proud, lazy, treacherous, thievish, hot, and addicted to all kinds of lusts, and most ready to promote them in others ... as ... revengeful, devourers of human flesh, and quaffers of human blood.... It is hardly possible to find in any African any quality but what is of the bad kind: they are inhuman, drunkards, deceitful, extremely covetous...." (cited in Fryer, 1984, p 153)

Further, he stated that there was a continuous chain of intellectual gradation from monkeys through varieties of black people, "until we mark its utmost limit of perfection in the pure white" (cited in Fryer, 1984, p 159).

William Knox, who had been provost-marshal of the British colony of Georgia in the mid-17th century, wrote one of the first openly racist pamphlets in Britain, in which he praised whipping black slaves, and justified treating them like 'brutes', when he stated that they were: "... a complete definition of indolent stupidity" and "... if they are incapable of feeling mentally, they will the more frequently be made to feel in their flesh" (cited in Fryer, 1984, p 159).

This has led contemporary academics such as Ramdin (1987) to argue that:

> Features such as hair and colour were the subsequent rationalisations to justify the simple economic fact that to fill the vacuum of colonial labour requirements, African labour was resorted to because it was cheapest and best. (Ramdin, 1987, p 4)

To planters during this period, black slaves were essentially a form of capital equipment, more easily and more cheaply replaceable than machinery (Fryer, 1988, p 14).

Notions of 'race', of biological superiority and inferiority, were expanded upon during the mid-19th century when there was the greatest migration of peoples in history, revealed in the mass migration of European immigrants to America, and to a lesser extent, Australia and South Africa (Hobsbawm, 1977). During this period, as a result of poverty, repression and famine in Ireland, there were high levels of Irish migration to Britain, when the Irish were described as, for example, "human chimpanzees", charged with "backwardness" (Curtis, 1984); notions of inferiority were based on the view that the Anglo-Saxon blood of the English was superior to the Celtic blood of the Irish (demonstrating that racism is not always an anti-black issue). Only a small minority of the population at the time, including members of the radical Chartist movement and the economist John Stuart Mill, saw that the poverty and violence in Ireland was the result not of Irish 'backwardness' but of British exploitation. In a pamphlet first published in 1834, the economist George Poulett Scrope urged the government to curb the nearly absolute powers of the landlords if it wished to avert starvation and revolution. It stated that:

> It is impossible … to have any doubt as to the real cause of the insurrectionary spirit and agrarian outrages of the Irish peasantry. They are the struggles of an oppressed starving people for existence!… They are the natural and necessary results of a state of law which allows the landlords of a country at one time to encourage an excessive growth of population on their estates, and at another, when caprice seizes them, to dispossess all this population, and turn them out on the highways without food and shelter. (cited in Curtis, 1984, p 50)

However, the most common explanation at the time, and one reflecting stereotypes used against the black population, was that the Irish,

> … hate our order, our civilisation, our enterprising industry, our sustained courage, our decorous liberty, our pure religion. This wild, reckless, indolent, uncertain and superstitious race has no sympathy with the English character. (Disraeli, 1836, cited in Curtis, 1984, p 51)

Labour migration patterns, caused by the expansion and development of capitalism in terms of both its demand for new labour and its effect in creating vast pools of poverty and misery among the dispossessed, were built on notions of 'race'. It bred division and reinforced inequalities within the social structure and was a process that was further reinforced by imperial expansion (Miles, 1982; Ramdin, 1987).

By 1914 the British Empire covered 12,700,000 square miles, with a population of 431 million, consisting of 370 million black people, but only 60 million of the white self-governing population. Britain's rulers therefore needed a racism more subtle and diversified, but just as aggressive, as that that was used to justify slavery (Fryer, 1988). As a result, from the 1840s to the 1940s, scientific theories reflecting notions of inferiority and superiority emerged to justify this exploitation. For example, phrenology, a pseudo-science that deduced people's characters from the shape of their skulls, was used to explain that the skulls of Africans clearly demonstrated their inferiority to humans. Anthropology was also used to demonstrate to the white British that black people were closer to apes than to Europeans, and that they were intellectually inferior, and social Darwinism that black people, as a result of their inferior intellect, were doomed to extinction. Racism was reinforced by the belief that God had fitted the British to rule over others – even though for most of human history Britain (and the North West of Europe generally) remained a remote and backward place, far behind the advanced societies of the Mediterranean, Indian continent and China (Harman, 1999). In its popular version, the message that black people were savages, who could be rescued from their 'barbaric and uncivilised' ways by British rule, was transmitted through schools, newspapers, literature and popular entertainment. The main political function of all these theories was to justify British rule over black people (Fryer, 1988).

Pseudo-scientific theories of 'race' developed to justify racism, slavery and imperial expansion. Yet there is no scientific basis for dividing the world's population into discrete, permanent, biological 'sub-species'. Scientific theories of 'race' have been disproved, and more recently, the science of genetics has confirmed this view by demonstrating that there is more statistically significant genetic diversity within population groups than between them (Miles and Phizacklea, 1984; Rose et al, 1984). The biologist Steven Rose (1984) claims:

> Where it has been possible to actually count up the frequencies of different forms of the genes and so get an objective estimate of genetic variation, 85 per cent turns out to be between individuals within the same local population, tribe, or nation; a further 8 per cent is between tribes or nations within a major 'race'; and the remaining 7 per cent is between major 'races'.... The remarkable feature of human evolution and history has been the very small degree of divergence between geographical populations as compared with genetic variation among individuals. (Rose et al, 1984, pp 126-7)

Thus 'race' is a social construct and not a scientifically valid concept. As Callinicos (1993) states:

> Racial differences are *invented*: that is, they emerge as part of a historically specific relationship of oppression in order to justify the existence of that relationship. So what is the historical peculiarity of racism as a form of oppression? In the first instance, it is that the characteristics which justify discrimination are held to be *inherent* in the oppressed group. A victim of racism can't change herself and thus avoid oppression; black people, for example, can't change their colour. This represents an important difference between, for example, racial and religious oppression, since one solution for someone persecuted on religious grounds is to change their faith. (Callinicos, 1993, p 18)

Nevertheless, despite the fact that scientific theories of racism have no validity, most people think that 'races' exist and institutions consciously and unconsciously discriminate against people on the grounds of 'race'. Thus while 'race' may not exist, racism certainly does. As Miles notes, racism is:

> ... an ideology which ascribes negatively evaluated characteristics in a deterministic manner ... to a group which is additionally identified as being in some way biologically ... distinct.... The possession of these supposed characteristics may be used to justify the denial of the group equal access to material and other resources and/or political rights. (Miles, 1982, pp 78-9)

As a consequence of socio-historical processes, racism is deeply embedded within capitalist social relations, it is part of the very structure of capitalist society and it is reflected in the practices of organisations and institutions operating within these societies (Miles, 1982; Fryer, 1984; Callinicos, 1993). Racism therefore remains a dominant feature of British society, and ideas reflecting notions of racial inferiority and superiority are still reproduced and reinforced in the labour market, the political arena, and within state institutions.

Postwar migration

In the postwar period, Britain experienced an acute labour shortage, and politicians actively sought labour from Commonwealth countries. As a result, during the 1950s and 1960s, economic migrants from Britain's Commonwealth entered the country because of the demands of the job market, and as a result of poverty and lack of opportunity in their country of birth (due to the immiseration of the colonies under the British Empire) (Castles and Miller, 1993; Miles, 1993; Wrench and Solomos, 1993). Workers were particularly needed in sectors of the economy characterised by the poorest pay and conditions, such as textiles, catering and public transport, which white workers could afford to reject in an era of economic expansion and full employment. But precisely because of the history of racism and the way it was deeply embedded within British society, migrants arrived to face harrowing levels of discrimination and abuse (Rex and Moore, 1967; The Runnymede Trust and the Radical Statistics Race Group, 1980). This is very important in understanding the position that the black population came to occupy both geographically and economically in Britain. The location of the black workforce within already overcrowded conurbations where they occupied the largely unskilled and low status jobs resulted in their also occupying very poor housing in inner-city areas. It also contributed to, and reinforced notions of, white superiority, for racism offered white workers the comfort of believing themselves to be superior to black workers, and during economic crises enabled employers and politicians to scapegoat black workers and blame them when levels of unemployment rose. From the 1940s onwards, the emergence of black communities in Britain has been shaped by the market forces of labour supply and demand, and therefore:

> ... suffused through every aspect of the influx and settlement of black persons is the exploitative relation between white and black characteristic in British history. (Husband, 1980, p 70)

The racism which black people experienced on their arrival in postwar Britain not only affected their entry to the labour market, but their access to other areas of social provision, and it also acted as a barrier to their involvement in British social life (Rex and Moore, 1967; Rex, 1973; Rex and Tomlinson, 1979). Most graphically, in Notting Hill and Nottingham in 1958 black people found themselves under violent attack from racists mobs. Under these circumstances migration became 'racialised' and increasingly viewed as a 'problem' (Miles and Phizacklea 1984)

During the 1960s and 1970s, Britain's black population continued to be located in low paid sectors of the economy, were more susceptible to unemployment, and experienced disproportionate levels of poverty (Fryer, 1984). However, their experiences worsened substantially from the 1970s onwards, when they bore the brunt of increasing poverty and inequality arising from economic recession and a political agenda that set out to demonise the poor and attack state benefits (Jones, 1998). Oppenheim (1993) stated that:

> In spite of government concern with racial disadvantage, and the undoubted limited success of positive action and equal opportunities in helping to create a black middle class, the condition of the black poor is deteriorating. (Oppenheim, 1993, p 115)

And Sivanandan (1998) argues that despite legislation to combat 'racial discrimination',

> ... in deprived and inner-city areas, on the dilapidated housing estates, in that third of society which has been socially and economically excluded for almost a generation, racism has got worse. There, racial attacks are on the increase, racial harassment is commonplace, and fascism finds ready recruits.... (Sivanandan, 1998, p 73)

However, despite the increasing deprivation they were facing, the black population were being blamed for rising levels of unemployment, revealing how, in times of economic crisis, governments still scapegoat the black population in order to detract from structural explanations of poverty and disadvantage. Sklar describes how:

> Racist and sexist scapegoating makes it easier to forget that the majority of poor people are white.... Many white men who are 'falling down' the economic ladder, are being encouraged to believe they are failing because women and people of colour are climbing over them to the top or dragging them down from the bottom. That way they will blame ... people of colour rather than the system. (cited in Jones, 1998, p 22)

From the 1950s to the 1980s, racist hostility was mainly directed towards Afro-Caribbean and Asian populations. However, it has now begun to shift onto new groups such as Roman gypsies and Albanians, utilising all the negative stereotypes formerly employed against the black population. For example, in Britain and across Europe there have been increasing attacks on immigration and the 'right to asylum', with officials and politicians depicting poor and vulnerable people as opportunists seeking to exploit the benefits of life within the European Union. These attacks, however, have been mainly launched against black, non-European migrants, who have been referred to as a 'threat', a 'population bomb' and a 'time bomb' (Lister, 1997, p 101).

The racialisation of British politics

The growth of black migration to Britain in the immediate postwar period provoked a series of racist responses. One was the development of state immigration controls whose aim was to limit black entry to Britain. Race-related legislation from the 1960s onwards demonstrates how the migration of labour to Britain has become increasingly tangled up in the politics of 'race'. It also reveals that racism, as well as being a consequence of economic conditions, is also mediated by the role played by politicians. For example, whereas politicians such as Enoch Powell encouraged black migration when there was a shortage of labour in the British economy, in later years he warned the British population that as a result of increased immigration:

> ... their wives [were] unable to obtain hospital beds on childbirth, their children were unable to obtain school places, their homes and neighbourhoods were changed beyond recognition. (cited in Sivanandan, 1981, p 82)

In the postwar period racial discrimination was legal, and employers and other groups such as landlords could simply state that 'no coloureds' were wanted. In the mid–1960s, in an atmosphere of increasing racist political activity, the government responded by adopting two related strategies: integration and restriction. Integration was to be achieved through a number of policies to promote appropriate relations between the 'races'. In 1965, the Race Relations Act made it unlawful to discriminate on the grounds of race, colour or ethnic or national origin in public places such as hotels, restaurants and swimming pools. The Act also set up the Race Relations Board to receive complaints of discrimination. Three years later, the Race Relations Act of 1968 made discrimination in the area of employment, housing and the provision of goods and services unlawful, and made it possible to bring cases of discrimination to court. The 1976 Race Relations Act replaced the 1968 Act, and for the first time the law was extended to cover indirect discrimination. That is, unlawful practices whatever their intentions, were shown to have a disproportionately adverse effect on the minority ethnic communities. The Commission for Racial Equality replaced the functions of the Race Relations Board at this juncture. A further piece of relevant legislation was the 1966 Local Government Act, which provided funds for what became known as 'Section 11' workers, who were employed to promote the integration of New Commonwealth immigrants into British society in areas such as education.

The second strand of government strategy was 'restriction' of black entry to Britain. In 1962 the Conservative government introduced the Commonwealth Immigrants Act which limited entry from the 'coloured' Commonwealth by making workers apply for different categories of work vouchers based on their occupational skills. Although the Labour government bitterly opposed this while in office, the degree of popular support for the measure caused serious problems for them during the

1964 election, and they reversed their position. They not only kept the Act on the statute books, but passed another such act in 1968 at the time of Enoch Powell's notorious speech on 'race' matters, and the crisis caused by the expulsion of British passport-holding Asians from Kenya (Penketh and Ali, 1997). In 1971 The Conservative government further tightened restriction on black migration by passing the Immigration Act, the consequence of which was that British passport holders from the New Commonwealth were no longer guaranteed entry to Britain. As Miles and Phizacklea (1984) note, the progressive tightening of entry requirements had a clear political implication: the black presence was viewed as creating political and social problems and the solution was to limit the numbers entering the country.

Since the 1980s, legislation associated with 'race' and immigration has become increasingly punitive as a result of economic recession, rising levels of unemployment, and the election of a Right-wing Conservative government who reinforced notions that the black British presence was a threat to Englishness or Britishness. This was reflected in the 1981 British Nationality Act, and by Margaret Thatcher's positive references to Britain's history as an imperial power. For example, in 1978 she stated that:

> ... you know, the British character has done so much for democracy, for law, and done so much throughout the world, that if there is a fear that it might be swamped, people are going to react and be rather hostile to those coming in. (cited in Miles, 1993, p 76)

But it is not just black migration that is viewed as 'problematic'. In the context of increasing global instability, the growth of oppressive regimes, and an escalation of internal conflict in areas such as the Balkans, the debate over immigration has now been expanded and applied to groups such as Kosovan refugees. These groups face the same direct and indirect abuse that Asian and Afro-Caribbean migrants faced in the past, portrayed as 'economic migrants' seeking to abuse the hospitality of European states, a view reinforced by politicians and sections of the press. For example, Michael Howard, the then Conservative Home Secretary, stated that:

> We are seen as a very attractive destination because of the ease with which people can gain access to jobs and benefits ... only a tiny proportion [of asylum seekers] are genuine refugees. (cited in Cook, 1998, p 152)

There is little or no recognition that refugees and asylum seekers have fled their home countries as a result of ethnic cleansing and/or repression, torture and death threats. As a result, legislation such as the Asylum and Immigration Act (1996), instead of focusing on the legal and welfare rights of immigrants, is increasingly involved in criminalising them (Cook, 1998).

Despite the claims of politicians regarding the generosity of the British welfare state, in reality the rights of immigrants and asylum seekers have been seriously curtailed in recent years. For example, under the 'no recourse to public funds' clause, immigrants are not entitled to a variety of state benefits, and their sponsors have to sign a declaration to that effect (Joint Council for the Welfare of Immigrants, 1995), and recommendations enshrined in the Asylum and Immigration Act (1996) have been criticised as criminalising and impoverishing asylum seekers and their families.

The 1996 Act has included withdrawing asylum seekers' rights to Income Support, child benefits, and public housing, and anyone not satisfying entry clearance requirements is liable to detention. Suspected immigration 'offenders' and asylum detainees may be held in police cells, and there is increasing evidence that incarceration is being used as a first rather than a last resort. Groups such as Amnesty International and the United Nations High Commission for Refugees have criticised the Act for the way it is administered, often by personnel of a low rank who are not subject to any independent scrutiny (Cook, 1998), and for the increased emotional stress it is imposing on groups who are already traumatised due to their past experiences and separation from their homes and families. Yet despite these concerns and criticisms, refugees have been attacked by sections of the British press and have been described as "scum of the earth" and "human sewage" (Marfleet, 1999, p 75), and by the mid-1990s, a network of prison camps and holding establishments had been set up across the European Union, with the British state imprisoning asylum seekers at a rate of 10,000 a year (*The Independent*, 28 June, 1999).

The most recent government proposal, which has now been withdrawn, was that visitors to Britain from the Indian subcontinent were to be asked to provide a £10,000 bond if they were suspected of planning to settle illegally in Britain. In a pilot scheme which was expected to begin in the autumn of 2000, British visa offices in India, Pakistan and Bangladesh were to require a financial guarantee before granting entry permission to visitors regarded as 'borderline' cases (Woodward, 2000), despite the fact that they make up only 5% of overseas entries. The money, which could be provided by family members, would be returned if visitors left the country on or before the date they were due to go. The proposal was criticised as branding all visitors from the Indian subcontinent as potential illegal immigrants. It seemed unlikely that the bond scheme would be applied to white visitors, despite the fact that together they account for 50% of all (non–EU national) visits to the United Kingdom each year.

That this is likely to be the case is borne out in evidence and statistics which reveal a clear class division at operation within the structure of racist exclusion (Miles, 1993). For example, during the early 1990s British passports were being offered legally to Hong Kong businessmen for £60,000, and the government's own immigration statistics show that, in 1998, the refusal rate for US citizens applying for visas to settle in Britain (almost all on the basis of being family members of a British resident) was only one for every 243 successful applications (less than 0.25%). Yet, Bangladeshi would-be settlers endured a refusal rate of around one in every three successful applications. There are also differential experiences among those intending to take holiday vacations and other trips that involve residence in Britain for less than six months. In 1998, there were eight million visitors in this category. Around one third were US citizens, with Japanese and Canadian citizens forming the next largest category, and of the 2.5 million US citizens in this category, only 0.04% were refused entry. However, Africans and peoples from the Indian subcontinent were required to obtain entry clearance before embarking on their journeys, and the refusal rate for visas was about 30% (*The Guardian*, 20 October, 1999).

The debate regarding immigration and asylum sets to continue and intensify. William Hague has identified it as one of the key 'battle grounds' in the next general election and the Conservative Party and the press are already orchestrating a campaign of hostility and discrimination. For example, *The Sun* (16 January 2000) ran a headline that read '10,000 Refugees in Queue to Live Here ... 264,000 Patients in Queue for NHS Beds'.

The tone of political and public debate regarding refugees and asylum seekers has been strongly criticised by Nick Hardwick, Chief Executive of the Refugee Council, who believes that Britain needs to take the crisis out of the asylum system. He recently stated that:

> It beggars belief that one of the richest countries in the world cannot deal with the tiny proportion of refugees who come to us without

becoming hysterical. We all have a responsibility to restore some sanity to the situation. (*The Guardian*, 11 February, 2000)

The Observer editorial (13 February, 2000) also expressed its disgust regarding the treatment of asylum seekers, when it stated that:

The widespread view is that Britain is a soft target for asylum seekers. The truth is different. Britain has so tightened up its asylum rules that the country is effectively impenetrable, with among the lowest rates of asylum seekers in the West. The level of financial support is miniscule and the welfare state is so inadequate it hardly offers protection for native Britons, let alone asylum seekers.... People need to be desperate to leave the country of their birth; most asylum-seekers are *bona-fide* applicants fleeing from oppression.... And when they enter, we need to ensure that natural justice is applied. That their claim is genuine unless proved otherwise, and, if accepted, that they have every right to be treated as properly as we would if the same tragedy befell us. The implicit racism [in the coverage of asylum seekers] expressed last week from the floor of the Commons to the *Nine O'Clock News* disgraced and belittled us all. (*The Observer*, 13 February 2000)

This is evidence of the continuing hold of racism, and the extent to which structural and institutional racism is embedded in British society. But the racialisation processes have another equally worrying side-effect. The drift of state policy increasingly to tighten entry requirements and problematise black immigration and asylum seekers allows distasteful proponents of far Right views to promote their politics and gain an apparent legitimacy. As Miles and Phizacklea (1984) note, the racialisation of politics and immigration policy has allowed fascist and nazi parties to seem 'respectable' as they engage with debate set by government discourse: if the problem is the black presence, if restriction on their entry is legitimate, then is repatriation so outrageous? Rather than seeing the problem as being the racism embedded in British society, the 'numbers game' played by politicians and the racialisation of politics have given the impression that it is the black presence which is a political and social problem. Such attitudes have also affected responses to the problem of racism.

Anti-discriminatory perspectives

The level of racism in British society has also produced various attempts to control or manage the situation. For some, this has been a problem of regulating relations between 'races'. Others have promoted socio-democratic notions of multiculturalism, while a minority current has been motivated by anti–racism. It is to these competing perspectives that I now turn.

Before offering a critical analysis of these perspectives it is worth noting that, despite their deficiencies and defects, they did represent a break from the violent and brutalising racism that had historically been evident, and they did, for the first time, allow some notion of black people as human beings. They also gave black communities in Britain an opportunity to present their traditions and cultures as something worthy of positive attention, and although the opportunities they presented were limited and conditional, many sections of the black population did respond enthusiastically to them. However, 'race relations' legislation and assimilationist perspectives were always built on the assumption that black and white people could not easily live together, and that education and tolerance went hand in hand with a restriction on immigration. Their inadequacies have been revealed, not by their theoretical or ideological analysis, but by their failure to make any fundamental difference to the 'social condition' of black people in British society. For example, black groups could give cookery demonstrations or entertain by playing in steel bands, but they were still discriminated against in the labour market, the housing market and in terms of educational provision (Institute of Race Relations, 1980; MacDonald et al, 1989).

Assimilationist/integrationist perspectives

Assimilationist perspectives are based on the belief in the cultural and racial superiority of white society and the associated belief that black groups should be absorbed into the indigenous homogenous culture. That is, they are expected to adopt the British 'way of life' and not to undermine the social and ideological bases of the dominant culture. Integrationist perspectives also subscribe to assumptions of cultural superiority, and therefore place the responsibility on black communities to learn 'new customs' and ways of behaving in order to be accepted by the indigenous population. However, they also believe that there has to be some attempt on the part of the 'host' community to understand the difficulties faced by black groups. Integration was described by Roy Jenkins in 1966 as "equal opportunity accompanied by cultural diversity in an atmosphere of mutual tolerance" (quoted in Troyna, 1992, p 68). However, both these 'race-related' perspectives, which still exert an influence today, tend to ignore the fact that most black people are British born and therefore quite competent in negotiating the dominant culture. For example, research carried out by HMSO (1994) revealed that 75% of the British black population are UK born, and at least a quarter of a million are of 'mixed race'.

Multiculturalism

During the 1970s and 1980s, 'multiculturalism' was reflected in government initiatives associated with 'race'. Multicultural perspectives are based on the notion that learning about other peoples' cultures will reduce prejudice and discrimination in society, and are mainly about 'doing' things such as celebrating cultural diversity within a theoretical framework which is informed by integrationist perspectives. They incorporate the belief that contact with other cultural lifestyles will reduce the ignorance and prejudice of the white population. However, they can be criticised for focusing on individualistic and cultural analyses rather than structural analyses to explain the discrimination which black people experience in society. As such, they fail to explain how and why black groups are disadvantaged. As Sivanandan stated:

> There is nothing wrong about learning about other cultures, but it must be said that to learn about other cultures is not to learn about the racism of your own ... unless you are mindful of the racial superiority inculcated in you by 500 years of colonisation and slavery, you cannot come to cultures objectively. (Sivanandan, 1991, p 41)

Analyses based on individuals and cultures led to the development of Racial Awareness Training (RAT) within state organisations, whose aim was to challenge racism by enabling professionals to 'discover' their personal racism. The implications of theorising racism as prejudice were criticised by Husband (1991), who stated that it:

> ... reduces racism to human nature and individual fallibility, thus leaving the world of the state, the world of politics and major structural aspects of contemporary life out of focus. (Husband, 1991, p 50)

The implementation of RAT not only reinforced the view that tackling individual prejudice was the major route to eliminating discrimination within professional institutions, but also had a tendency to intensify the defensiveness and guilt that white professionals experienced around issues of 'race' and racism. Thus, although it represented a significant change in seeking not to pathologise black people, it created an atmosphere that made many professionals wary of subsequent anti-racist initiatives.

Despite the flaws inherent in these 'race-related' initiatives informed by cultural pluralism, they dominated the political agenda throughout the 1970s, until the election of Margaret Thatcher in 1979 who wanted to dismantle all 'race-relations' legislation and multicultural programmes (Saggar, 1992). Despite the Conservative Party's commitments, however, as the 1980s progressed they utilised a range of 'race-related' initiatives. This was a result of uprisings in black communities. "The most significant were those in Bristol in 1980, in London, Liverpool, Manchester and other towns in 1981, in Birmingham, Bristol, London, Liverpool and various other towns in 1985" (Hasan, 2000, p 173). Conservative politicians revived Section 11 funding (specialist funding to support local government initiatives aimed at promoting the 'integration' of the black community) and promoted 'equal opportunities', often by putting black people in bureaucratic positions of power which, for some, led to their alienation from the black community. For example, Sivanandan (1982) stated:

> All the system did was make more room for the rising black petty-bourgeoisie – to get them into the media, the police force, local government, parliamentarise them – to deter extra-parliamentary protests. (Sivanandan, 1982, p ii)

He argued that such development operated in such a way as to obstruct any latently political programme, and that the emergence of a black bourgeoisie who worked with the state took the politics out of black struggles. This enabled the development of reformist anti-racism that emphasised government action at the expense of real change, and although it won over middle-class black people and the white metropolitan Left (both significant in terms of CCETSW's developments; see Chapter Three), it left racism untouched. It also led to funding policies introduced by, for example, the Greater London Council and other Left-led councils in the early 1980s, which had a tendency to place groups such as Asians, Africans and Caribbeans, in competitive relationships with each other. Davidson (1999) has also commented that:

> When social change is destructive of established ways of life, and class politics does not offer an alternative, then group membership may seem the only way of scavaging what you can in the struggle over resources. This is reinforced when the left focuses on the myths of ethnicity, and refuses to accept that 'identity' can never be irrelevant or simply a cover for sectional interests. (Davidson, 1999, p 13)

It was during the early 1980s, as a response to the Brixton riots, that the Scarman Report was published. The report denied the existence of institutional racism. Instead, it defined racism as individual prejudice. Not surprisingly, it was well received by superiors within the police force, reflecting their belief that the problem was one of a few 'rotten apples in the force' rather than a 'rotten barrel' (Barker and Beazer, 1983; Sivanandan, 1990). Furthermore, the police claimed that the behaviour of officers was itself occasioned by the street culture of black youth, "spending much of their lives on the streets ... are bound to come into contact with criminals and the police". Police 'misconduct' was then blown out of all proportion into a "myth of brutality and racism" by the "West Indian habit of rumour-mongering and their flair for endless discussion of ... grievances" (cited in Sivanandan, 1982, p i).

In defence of anti-racism

In the late 1970s and early 1980s anti-racist perspectives began to emerge, which in contrast to previous policies based on assimilationist/ integrationist and multiculturalist perspectives, went beyond a concern with individual prejudice and culture in order to expose the structural and institutional nature of racism in society. This perspective was supported by a major survey published in 1984 by the Policy Studies Institute on the position of black people in Britain. It demonstrated that black people were still generally employed below their qualifications and skill levels, earned less than white workers in comparable jobs, and were still concentrated in the same industries as they were 25 years earlier (Brown, 1984). It also revealed discrimination in areas of welfare provision such as housing and education.

Anti-racist perspectives offer a much more radical interpretation of discrimination within society. The historical and social construction of 'race' and racism, discussed earlier, emphasises the ways in which racism has developed in relation to the expansion of slavery, imperialism and migration. The state, and a range of state institutions, have played crucial roles in disseminating and mediating 'race' and racialisation processes. Thus, anti-racist perspectives point to the ways in which racism is built into the structures and institutions of capitalist society. Thus, they are sceptical about the extent to which legislative reform alone can successfully challenge racism, or improve the lives of the black population. These doubts reflect a belief that the state is not neutral or independent, but is an expression of an economic, social and political system that benefits from racism by oppressing black people and dividing workers along racial lines – that it is a structural and institutional phenomenon within capitalist societies.

Consequently, strategies to tackle racism have involved external challenges by anti-racist organisations and coalitions within the communities, the workplace, and within state institutions. For many anti-racists the fight against racism must be left to the black community itself, but this would seem to limit the potential power and mobilising effects that anti-racist struggles can generate. Over the last 20 years in Britain there have been a number of important examples of black and white groups standing together to defeat racist policies and practices, and to confront racist organisations. For example, in the mid-1970s the Grunwick's strike led by Asian (mainly women) workers, became a central focus for the working-class movement at the time. The predominantly Asian workforce was supported by a series of mass pickets of overwhelmingly white trade unionists, and the factory was 'blacked' by local post workers (Ramdin, 1987). In the late 1970s 'Rock Against Racism' and the Anti-Nazi League were able to mobilise large numbers of black and white youth and various political activists in the struggle against both racism and the far-Right (Jenkins, forthcoming). In a series of uprisings in the 1980s and 1990s, black, Asian and white youth fought together against poverty, deprivation and state policing (Hasan, 2000), while more recently, in 1999 at the Ford plant in Dagenham, an overwhelmingly white workforce went on strike against racism meted out to black workers by supervisors, and the struggle of the Lawrence family was supported by various trade unionists such as firefighters, postal workers and council workers. This led black writer, Darcus Howe, to comment that there had been greater solidarity for the family from the white working class than the black middle class (Ferguson and Lavalette, 1999).

Anti-racist activity has also been evident in other parts of Europe.

For example, in the 1990s in France there were massive mobilisations of black and white youth demonstrating against racist attacks, and in Paris in 1997 there was a demonstration attended by large contingents of anti-fascists from other European countries that attracted 100,000 protesters (Marfleet, 1999). On 19 February 2000, there was a demonstration of over 300,000 people, protesting against the inclusion of the fascist Freedom Party within the Austrian government, a protest that included black and white people from across Europe. These and similar events are often ignored or dismissed within the anti-racist literature (see Ramdin, 1987 and Gilroy, 1987), but, for reasons which will be discussed in the following section, they remain important occasions which demonstrate the possibility and potential of black and white unity in the anti-racist struggle.

The politics of identity

Anti-racist strategies, with their focus on structural and institutional racism, had varying degrees of success in challenging racism in British society, and were linked to a movement that was successful in preventing the growth of far-Right, nazi organisations such as the National Front in parts of Britain. However, during the 1980s, as the political climate moved rightwards, the various movements spurned by the 'explosion' of 1968 went into retreat and moved towards more constitutional forms of politics. This was reflected in the academy when the '68 generation' moved towards a variety of post-modernist theories about the shape and form of the modern world (Callinicos, 1989).

Post-modernist ideas are not easily defined as many of their chief proponents disagree on their meaning, but their key elements "... stress the fragmentary, heterogeneous and plural character of reality" (Smith, 1994, p 5). As Ferguson and Lavalette (1999) have argued, elements of post-modern theorising have been important in shaping a politics based on identity. Here the concepts of 'identity' and 'difference' have increasingly replaced that of 'oppression' in discussions relating to the social position of minority groups in society. Yet while 'oppression' tends to be associated with the practices of 'racism', 'patriarchy' or the material inequalities of capitalism or its social relations, 'identities', by contrast, are viewed as free-floating and fluid, and even a matter of choice. Kath Woodward, for example, suggests:

> Discourses, whatever sets of meanings they construct, can only be
> effective if they recruit subjects. Subjects are thus subjected to the

discourse and must themselves take it up as individuals who so position themselves. The positions which we take up and identify with constitute our identities. (Woodward, 1997, p 39)

Woodward further suggests that identity politics "involves claiming one's identity as a member of [a] ... marginalized group as a political point of departure" (Woodward, 1997, p 24).

These passages suggest that identity is first and foremost a matter of choice. An identity is chosen – for example, as a black woman, a gay man, an environmental activist – in the same way that a lifestyle is chosen. But while some sections of society may be able to make such choices, for the vast majority (and perhaps especially those who come into contact with the local social work department) the identities on offer are few in number, often undesirable and imposed by the state. Few would choose the identities of social work client or unemployed claimant, for example.

Second, dissolving any link between identities and social structures, and the promotion of a 'celebration of difference', can trivialise oppression. As Smith argues:

> In place of systematic analysis we are given impressionism. By this method, oppression is something which is self-articulated and self-defined, having no objective basis in larger society. This approach can and does result in trivialising genuine human suffering – by lumping it together with all in society who define themselves as 'oppressed' – such as middle-class consumers and anti-authoritarian or counter-cultural middle-class youth, whose complaints may be valid, but who hardly constitute specially oppressed groups in society. (Smith, 1994, p 29)

Callinicos (1995) argues that there is nothing inherently progressive about identity politics, a point borne out perhaps by the various ethnic conflicts in the Balkans and various other parts of the globe, each of which is in no small part concerned about issues of identity. But, he continues, "even in its 'radical variants', [identity politics] is vulnerable to the most serious historical, philosophical and political criticism" (Callinicos, 1995, p 198). These criticisms include their regular dependence on 'invented traditions', the fact that specific identities are "typically constituted in contrast and sometimes opposition to other identities" and that it leads to a politics of fragmentation (Callinicos, 1995, p 198).

Expanding these themes, Benhabib (1995) has warned that identity politics has led to the 'Balkanisation' of urban America, which has seen various groups using their 'identities' as a justification in their competition for jobs, housing and various education and welfare benefits. Todd Gitlin has suggested that the current obsession with difference is marginalising that "frame of understanding and reference that understands 'difference' against a background of what is not different, what is shared among groups" (Gitlin, 1994, p 144). While Johnson (2000) argues that:

> ... particularistic social policy is inescapably divisive, not because it accepts the reality of diverse needs, but because, in essentialising each group or identity and positioning each in a unilateral relationship to the state as a client, it detaches social policy from any ethic of solidarity and therefore from any possibility of systemic social change, and so risks replicating rather than rupturing the ugly and unequal textures of capitalist society. (Johnson, 2000, p 101)

These issues have been taken up by some black writers in Britain who criticise 'identity politics' and the 'right to be different' for usurping the 'right to be equal', and for accepting rather than challenging societal divisions and inequalities (Malik, 1996).

In contrast to anti-racist perspectives, identity politics marginalises explanations based on economic and political analyses, and does not offer an adequate understanding of the material hardship and deprivation which black people face. The focus on cultural resistance and 'ethnic difference' also conceals class antagonisms within the black 'community'. For example, the housing needs of a working-class Asian living in run down, overcrowded accommodation are not the same as for a middle-class Asian living in the suburbs. In short, while a stress on culture may be informative, and provide an important boost to anti-racism, it cannot confront the material realities of class rule, and black liberation cannot come from non-work-based cultural activities.

In recent years the growing hold of a politics of identity among anti-racist writers has meant that the term 'black' has been replaced with a series of terms, each apparently more attuned to the cultural identities of various minority ethnic communities. Modood claimed that the term 'black' sold short the majority of the people it defined in this way (Modood, 1988, p 397) (although it is unlikely that replacing 'black' by some other politically neutral description will secure a more equitable distribution of resources). But it is unclear to what extent this new 'sensitivity' towards issues of identity and cultural specificity is accepted within minority communities in Britain. For example, the Bradford Commission Report in 1996 cites an Asian man defining his communities as follows:

> I would view myself as a member of the following communities, depending on the context and in no particular order: Black, Asian, Azad Kashmiri, Kashmiri, Mirpuri, Jat, Maril'ail, Kungriwalay, Pakistani, English, British, Yorkshireman, Bradfordian, from Bradford Moor.... I could use the term 'community' in any of these contexts and it could have meaning. Any attempt to define me as only one of these would be meaningless. (Bradford Commission, 1996, p 92)

In contrast, radical activists involved in fighting racism adopted the term 'black' in the late 1960s. They used the term to reflect a unifying and universal politics of solidarity that was mobilised as part of a set of ideas and principles promoting collective action. Interestingly, among many of the 'family campaigns' (that is, those campaigns run by the families of various victims of racist violence and murder, such as the Lawrences and the Reels), the term 'black' has been adopted consciously to emphasise the commonality of their oppression. It is for these reasons that the term 'black' will be used throughout the rest of the book.

CCETSW's anti-racist initiative

The previous sections have discussed and analysed the concepts of 'race' and racism, how racism emerged in a specific economic context, and how it is reproduced and reinforced in contemporary society. An historical analysis of British legislative developments reveals that 'race-related' policies have never seriously addressed the structural and institutional manifestation of racism in British society. Instead, policies have reflected a political agenda concerned to restrict or prohibit (mainly black) immigration. Strategies to deal with racism within state welfare institutions have mainly reflected perspectives associated with assimilation and integration of the black community, or enhancing cultural awareness. But, CCETSW's anti-racist initiative was concerned with tackling institutional racism, reflecting the belief that racism is endemic in British society, and reproduced within state institutions. CCETSW's Paper 30 supported a policy agenda that would deal with the institutional manifestation of racism, but it was subject to a fundamental backlash and a denial that institutional racism was a feature of the social work profession.

Using CCETSW's anti-racist initiative as a case study, this book explores why challenges to institutional racism within state organisations face such hostility. It will do this by analysing the development and implementation of CCETSW's anti-racist programme as a 'top-down' anti-discriminatory policy initiative. That is, an initiative which sought to alter the conditions of social work activity by imposing directive and prescribed forms of behaviour and practice 'from above' onto students, academics, workers and professionals in the field. Of course, all social policy initiatives in this sense reflect 'top-down' approaches to social change, and all are attempting to engineer a particular outcome. But CCETSW's policy initiative was unusual in that it reflected an anti-racist perspective that signified a move beyond policies associated with multiculturalist, 'culturally sensitive' or 'culturally aware' approaches. Instead it incorporated a theoretical recognition that Britain is a structurally and institutionally racist society, and attempted to implement a 'top-down' initiative promoting a 'progressive policy of anti-racism'. Further, it assumed that academic establishments providing social work education, and social work agencies themselves, were institutionally racist. Thus it was intended that the policy would operate in conflictual, and to varying degrees, hostile environments, and would, in part, confront, challenge and engage with existing practices and policies regarding the treatment of both black workers and clients.

But the imposed policy failed to engage with, and win over, the majority of social work academics and practitioners. This failure left the initiative vulnerable to counterattacks from the media, politicians and those hostile within the profession. The book will therefore reveal both the possibilities and limits inherent in CCETSW's approach. Further, although Paper 30 was developed during the early 1990s, and was primarily concerned with social work education and training, it provides a useful and important case study of the possibilities, limitations and barriers facing critical and progressive policy initiatives in a range of institutions (welfare and non-welfare) in society today.

An analysis of CCETSW's developments will be based on research which was undertaken at the University of Central Lancashire between 1990 and 1992, which, in the context of CCETSW's anti-racist initiative, explored the implications for social work education and training by interviewing a number of black and white students and their respective practice teachers while they were on placement in social work agencies. This research revealed the institutional nature of racism within social work agencies, and demonstrated that, while anti-racist initiatives are clearly relevant to welfare organisations in a society structured by inequality, policy initiatives by themselves do not necessarily invoke change. That is, despite CCETSW's commitment to tackling institutional racism, as a 'top-down' policy initiative it was relatively limited in developing anti-racist practice within social work institutions which themselves operated in ways that reflected and embodied institutional racism. The backlash against Paper 30 was also evidence that 'top-down' policies are always vulnerable to counter-policies from political opponents hostile to anti-racist perspectives. To understand the basis of the professional opposition to Paper 30, it is necessary to look at the history of state social work, and the competing perspectives over the function and role of social work in modern society.

TWO

Social work, the state and society

CCETSW's Paper 30 was a brave and remarkable attempt to move beyond assimilationist and multicultural perspectives to challenge institutional racism within social work education, training and practice. However, its anti-racist initiative received a mixed response among practitioners who, as a group of professionals, do not share the same perspective regarding the role of social work in society. As Robert Pinker, an opponent of Paper 30, states:

> The possibility that staff and students might have ethical views of their own about such matters never seemed to concern the council. (Pinker, 1999, p 17)

In a sense, Pinker was right. Social work has always consisted of competing perspectives over, for example, its place within the welfare establishment, its attitude towards family values or the relative merits of its 'caring' and 'controlling' aspects. For ease of understanding, we can identify three broad perspectives concerning social work's role and function in society: 'conservative', 'social democratic' and 'radical'. Each of these offers a different analysis of the role of social work and its relationship with its mainly poor and disadvantaged client groups, and hence, I will suggest they were always likely to respond differently to various anti-discriminatory initiatives. In order to understand social work's response to CCETSW's anti-racist developments, it is necessary to analyse historically how the differing social work perspectives emerged, and their underlying assumptions.

The origins of social work

Social work developed in the context of both industrialisation and urbanisation. Industrialisation created new demands for labour and redefined the categories of people who could be seen as suitable workers, marginalising those who were not part of the labour market. It also produced problems of low-waged employment, and seasonal and cyclical unemployment, which gave rise to increasing poverty, and the expansion of cities and towns which led to problems of housing, ill health and unsanitary living conditions (Clarke, 1993). This produced an element of fear among the middle classes, who believed that such developments would give rise to disorder and disruption, especially as the capacity of the traditional charitable institutions to respond to need was diminished (Mooney, 1998). The reforms that emanated from these concerns were devoted to reinforcing an appropriate system of social values centering on thrift, sobriety, self-discipline and family life. Thus, by the end of the 19th century, there was a complex array of institutions to care for or reform a variety of people seen as constituting different types of social problems. For example, workhouses, prisons, asylums, schools and borstals were created to subject 'problem populations' to institutional regimes separate from the rest of society. At the same time there was a growth in the scientific classification of the human population that involved dividing, subdividing and categorising different sections of the population based on medical, biological and subsequently psychological sciences. These classifications governed how individuals were to be treated, how their 'progress' was to be measured and what principles should control their reform. A classification based on 'race' was also implemented, which identified racial types by bodily characteristics, mental capacities and emotional traits, used, for example, to justify the repression of the Irish and in constructing the Aliens Act to prevent the importation of 'foreign subversion' (in reality, to control and limit the entry of East European Jewish migrants fleeing pogroms in Poland and Russia) (Cohen, 1996). It also led to developments such as the introduction of school meals and medical inspections to improve the 'stock' and 'fitness' of the British 'race'. However, these measures were partly shaped by eugenicist theories which were concerned with controlling the 'eligibility to breed' of certain groups (Clarke, 1993).

The motivation behind voluntary activities and middle-class welfare intervention was characterised by a degree of compassion, but also by fear. Fear over the potentially destructive effects of social problems, and fear that charity would be exploited by groups not wanting to support themselves; these themes are still evident in the area of social services provision in Britain today. As a result, initiatives were developed which would establish personal contact between those administering and those receiving charitable provision, which enabled practical assistance in the form of what was to be termed 'casework', but which were also characterised by 'middle-class' moral judgements and values (Jones, 1983). For example, Charitable Organisation Society members worked alongside Poor Law guardians to separate the 'deserving' from the 'undeserving' poor, and to provide assistance that might help deserving cases to become independent (Steadman-Jones, 1971). Middle-class women who reflected the assumptions and 'norms' of middle-class life, and whose involvement with working-class women centred on issues associated with childcare and the family, also dominated voluntary activity. Consequently, issues of morality rather than structural issues of power, employment or marginalisation characterised intervention and affected judgements. These, then, were the areas of social intervention that formed the origins of social work in Britain, which were characterised by a dialectic of care and control. Social workers offered personalised assistance to individuals often suffering the most extreme forms of hardship, but in a way that allowed them to evaluate, direct and make decisions about clients' lives, and which involved making character evaluations regarding the appropriateness of their lifestyles, manners and habits. In this respect they distinguished between the deserving and undeserving poor, and perceived social problems in an individualised way. For example, when the School of Sociology was founded by the Charitable Organisation Society in 1902, for knowledge to be deemed relevant and acceptable it had to support the "primacy of individualism and endorse the prevailing social order" (Jones, 1996, p 192).

Early proponents of social work, who viewed social reform as a political danger that could undermine social order, were able to distinguish their approach from reform or socialism. Milnes stated:

> Casework then, becomes the antithesis of mass or socialistic measures, and the defender of casework finds that his plan will not rest merely on negating socialism, but in proving that there is still much to be said for what can be described as individualism. (cited in Walton, 1975, p 150)

As a result, conventional social norms about, for example, work, the family, and the care of children, were replicated within the theories and orientations of social work, and tended to incorporate the reproduction of social divisions and forms of inequality. This does not infer that all social workers lack compassion, care and concern, or that clients have not been helped by social work intervention, but offers an important recognition that as a form of social intervention, social work was dominated by pressures to separate the alleviation of individual misery from concerns with structural inequality. As the welfare activities of both national and local government expanded during the interwar years, elements of social work began to be drawn into the operations of the state, and in 1936, the British Federation of Social Workers was formed to create some sense of unity out of the diverse conditions of social work. However, even in the context of the development of more collective measures, social work was promoted as having a distinctive concern with, and sensitivity to, the individual that was lacking in other areas of welfare intervention, and the predominant focus of theory and practice was around family relationships. Thus, the conservatism of social work's core knowledge base persisted in the context of the birth of the post-1945 social democratic welfare state, when the social work curricula included those aspects of sociology which, according to Leonard, "reinforced and supported the reformist and familial domain assumptions of social work" (cited in Jones, 1996, p 195).

The emergence of state social work

As social work as a profession developed during the 1960s, the role of social workers began to reflect the social democratic concerns of the era, inherent in the Seebohm Report (1968). There was a political commitment to enhancing social citizenship through promoting equality and solidarity, and social services departments were to "reach far beyond the discovery and rescue of social casualties" to "enable the greatest possible number of individuals to act reciprocally, giving and receiving service for the well-being of the whole community" (Seebohm, 1968, para 2). In this respect, there were attempts to redress residual social inequalities and to move away from the stigmatising and paternalistic traditions of voluntary welfare agencies.

Nevertheless, it is important to note that the Seebohm Report took an essentially optimistic view of social problems in Britain at that time. As Langan (1993) stated:

> It considered that conditions of post-war economic expansion sustained by political consensus and a comprehensive welfare state had largely eradicated the major structural problems of poverty, ignorance, disease, slum housing and mass unemployment, the 'five giants' identified in Beveridge's famous wartime report. (Langan, 1993, p 49)

It assumed that numbers in need of assistance were relatively small and that people's problems were characterised by a difficulty in adjusting to the complexities of modern life. Again, this assumption demonstrated the separation of personal problems from issues of material inequality.

The Seebohm Report was also contradictory, as it proclaimed a universalistic approach to counter the stigma of selectivism, while continuing to be preoccupied with 'problem families' and 'difficult personalities'. In this respect, social workers were still "selective benefactors of the modern equivalent of the deserving poor" (Langan, 1993, p 52). Critics of 'new' social democratic developments were concerned that in practice they identified "... emergent problems as minor internal malfunctions of the system requiring only further corrective technical strategies" (Clarke, 1980, p 179).

The political and professional optimism which marked the Seebohm Report was short-lived, as it was soon followed by a period of economic recession and political retrenchment in the 1970s. Social services departments came up against budgetary restrictions at the same time as changing social, economic and demographic patterns produced increasing demands for their services, and put added pressure on social workers. As Webb states:

> Any intention there may have been at the time of the Seebohm Report of producing a universal service to set alongside the National Health Service, has been destroyed by the twin forces of rising demand and public expenditure restraint which characterised the second half of the 1970s. Despite a few faltering steps towards a universal service, the personal social services have not fully escaped from the residual model of their Poor Law origins. (Webb, 1980, p 279)

Such developments led to a growing crisis of confidence among social workers, and the tension between their caring and controlling functions increased. Nevertheless, despite the persistence of individualistic and familial analyses in the field, broadly social democratic concerns became part of the dominant ideology of state social work activity – to deal with the worst manifestations of poverty and inequality, and to use the expanding welfare services to deal with the problems faced by the system's victims.

There have also been intermittent attempts by some in the profession to challenge structural inequalities in society, and to redefine their role as clients' advocates. During the 1970s, social work clients began challenging the legitimacy of social workers' definitions of their situation and needs, and at the same time the radical social work movement endorsed many of these criticisms and sought to transform the theory and practice of social work (Langan, 1993). The movement included a new generation of social workers who had been radicalised by wider trends in the student, labour and new social movements of the late 1960s and early 1970s. Radical social workers began to challenge social work's preoccupation with individualistic explanations of social problems which they condemned for pathologising the poor, and instead they developed analyses based on a mix of socialist, feminist and progressive political perspectives. The radical social work movement urged social workers to get involved in socialist political action in their own interests and the interests of their clients, demonstrating opposition to their controlling role in society.

However, as Clarke notes:

> Such efforts ... took place at the edges, rather than at the centre of social work, and in general terms, we might say that social work has tended to reproduce rather than redress social inequality. (Clarke, 1993, p 18)

Even in the context of more progressive social democratic welfare developments during the postwar period, social work retained its emphasis on individualising social problems and pathologising the poor, and it also continued to be characterised by tensions between its caring and controlling role in society. Further, social work, government agencies and politicians have always been concerned:

> ... to prevent social workers from being either radicalised or demoralised by their daily experiences of contact and involvement with some of the most deprived and impoverished sections of society. (Jones, 1996, p 191)

Jones (1996) suggests there are clear continuities within the dominant social work perspectives which tend to view clients as "generally unworthy and manipulative individuals" (p 197), while Kwhali asserts that:

> While the 'core values' of social work might arguably emphasise notions of justice, equity, empowerment and humanity, these concepts have seldom been actualised within the profession's own structures ... nor within its practice. Issues of control, containment, inequality and oppression are central not simply to the social workers' daily tasks, responsibilities and dilemmas, but to the wider organisational and societal contexts within which social work is located. (Kwhali, 1991, p 41)

Sivanandan (1991, p 31) went as far as claiming that in the Thatcherite era, social work became the 'new soft policing'. There has always been a gap between the theory and practice of social work. The 'core values' of social work, taught on courses and included in training, may reflect a social democratic image of society, but the institutionalised practices of social work departments are often reduced to a restrictive set of conservative assertions, made worse from the mid-1970s by the imposed restrictions of financial rectitude in an era of cuts.

Despite the fact that during the 1970s a more radical social work movement developed that challenged individualistic analyses informing social work intervention, social work practice has rarely been informed by structural analyses. Furthermore, political developments during the 1970s led Langan (1993) to observe pessimistically that:

> The social workers' strikes of the late 1970s and the election of a Conservative government on an aggressively anti-welfare programme in 1979 brought a miserable decade for social work to a grim conclusion. (Langan, 1993, p 62)

The new Right and social work developments

The treatment of clients and the status of professional social workers were further undermined during the 1980s and 1990s as a result of the various Conservative governments' policies influenced by an ideological commitment to removing minimal welfare protection for the poor and disadvantaged. This generally involved a reduction in public expenditure, a curb on welfare provision and the activities of local government, and the promotion of the private sector as a key player in the provision of social care (Johnson, 1990; Manthorpe and Stanley, 1997). These changes were indicative of the development of 'popular capitalism' that was characterised by the pursuit of possessive individualism, and an increasingly authoritarian definition of the national interest in moral and political affairs (Jessop et al, 1988).

In the context of financial cutbacks and a fundamental ideological attack on state welfare provision, social work staff began to experience the force of Conservative legislation. They were expected to respond to changes in the delivery and administration of social work provision in a climate of increasing poverty and deprivation, while being consistently attacked by the press, and having their professional credentials undermined. At the same time as the most oppressed and disadvantaged in society were being increasingly dehumanised and criminalised, social work was being criticised as too 'understanding' and not 'condemning' enough. This led to a re-examination of the nature of the skills required at the interface of client need and service provision. As a result, therapeutic social work intervention was undermined at the expense of an increase in regulation, surveillance and rationing. In the area of probation, for example, there was a complete restructuring of qualifying training during the 1990s, which led to a historic break with the Diploma in Social Work. Probation officer training has now been removed from its social work roots, thereby disbanding a system of training that had been painstakingly built up over a period of nearly a century (Williams, 1996). Novak (1995, p 8) claims, in relation to the subordination of education to work, that what is now offered is "a mechanical training in how to do the job and a rejection of the knowledge and understanding that is required to do it effectively". Webb (1996, p 179) added that the emphasis on training and specification of competencies had allowed "an intrusiveness into the academy that was hitherto not possible". CCETSW, in succumbing to new Right pressures to undermine the professional value base of social work, revealed their relative weakness to protect social work education. The government and many within the social work profession saw the review of the Diploma in Social Work (see below) as a triumph of 'common sense' over 'Left-wing politically correct ideology'. As Webb notes:

> Since its [CCETSW's] approach to anti-discrimination has been framed around competencies to the almost total exclusion of analysis and 'knowledge', it remains epistemologically unstable. By this I mean that anti-discrimination becomes precarious and easily eroded. (Webb, 1996, p 18)

The origins of social work remind us that it was never intended to be a practice which would remedy or reform structural inequality. Rather, it was about helping unfortunate people to help themselves, and was an explicit alternative to 'socialist' measures directed at more structural reform. In this respect social work can be seen as a peculiar and ambiguous practice which is concerned with human suffering, yet is set against changing social structures which might be causing this suffering. It is also a practice characterised by tensions, as social workers are expected to balance the needs of clients with the needs of society. To some extent this has been resolved by "assuming clients' needs and society's needs are the same: restoring the client to 'normal functioning' to satisfy everyone's interests" (Clarke, 1993, p 19).

But the history of social work development, and the various conceptions of social work's role in society, are not merely abstract theoretical issues; they filter through to practice where different practitioners have different political conceptions of their roles and responsibilities. In particular, it is possible to identify three broad models of social work practice: 'conservative', 'traditional social democratic' and 'radical'. These models reflect the three strains of ideas that have influenced British social work in the 20th century, and reflect different philosophies and practices in working with deprived and disadvantaged groups. The following section develops these models more fully.

Social work perspectives

Social workers are not a homogenous group who share the same philosophy regarding their professional role in working with client groups. Like the population as a whole, a range of ideas evident in class-divided societies influence them. These influences can be conceptualised as producing three broad models of social work practitioner.

Conservative professionals

The practice of social workers who could be termed 'conservative professionals' reflects the historical roots of social work as incorporated in the work of the Charity Organisation Society, for example. Accordingly, practitioners utilise notions of the 'deserving' and 'undeserving' poor in their work with different client groups, and their practice tends to be characterised by mechanisms of control. At the core of their values is a focus on a range of individualistic and familial theories that tend to pathologise poor client groups. A greater priority is given to the implementation of practical skills over education, especially with regard to any critical analysis enshrined in the social sciences, leading to an emphasis on 'practically' doing the job, as opposed to driving an agenda which 'uses clients' to justify social workers' political goals.

Social democratic workers

The second group could be termed 'social democratic' social workers. This is not intended to suggest an explicit commitment to any political party, but would reflect broad 'social democratic' concerns about society.

It includes a recognition that there are inherent inequalities in society, and that these have a detrimental impact on clients' lives. But there is the expectation that these can be solved, mainly by appropriate legislation, and, for example, intervention by welfare professionals. In this respect, they could be seen to reflect notions of justice and inequality, and a Fabian commitment to the possibility of progressive social engineering. However, there are contradictions in their philosophy. For example, they may be concerned about inequalities in society, yet at the same time reinforce discrimination by their support for the 'traditional' family structure and underlying gendered assumptions.

Radical social workers

Finally, there are social workers whose philosophy and practice could be termed 'radical'. This refers to a group of workers who have moved beyond the 'social democratic' consensus to embody a radical critique of social work intervention based on the recognition of fundamental structural inequalities evident in society. They move beyond individual and familial analyses to perceive social work clients as victims of social circumstances. In this respect, some radical social workers portray their position as being 'in and against' the state (Joyce et al, 1988). That is, although they view social workers generally as 'agents' of state social work, primarily geared to controlling and directing the poor, they consciously use their position within the state social work bureaucracy to obtain facilities and resources for the poor. They view themselves as being on the side of the poor and their primary concern is to protect them against exploitation. Issues of oppression based on class, gender and 'race', for example, are viewed as structural phenomena, and thus for these workers it is necessary that social workers understand and grasp the nature of these inequalities and oppressions if they are to have the knowledge base necessary to deal with their clients' problems. However, as Langan (1993) stated:

> Radical social work was always a minority movement and it lost momentum as the wider political left went into decline in the late 1970s. (Langan, 1993, p 60)

If we analyse these three groups in the abstract, in relation to issues of 'race' and anti-racist social work developments, we could suggest that 'conservative professionals' would be hostile to anti-discriminatory education, training and practice. This would be related to the fact that they tend to individualise and pathologise social problems, rather than analysing them in a structural context. The majority of social workers who encapsulate a 'social democratic' perspective would tend not to be overtly hostile to anti-discriminatory initiatives. As a perspective that recognises the 'social nature' of many societal problems, it is possible for adherents of this broad view to be convinced of the negative impact certain structural inequalities can produce. However, in the absence of committed anti-racist policies, education and training and an institutionally racist working environment, there would be a tendency to treat black clients no differently to white clients, leading to a 'race' blind approach to social work practice, to reduce anti-racism to (at best) a well-meaning multiculturalism. In contrast, the commitment of radical social workers to structural inequalities would result in this group being open and responsive to anti-racist developments, even in the face of institutionally racist assumptions and practice.

Although these three groups represent an 'ideal type', they are useful in identifying perspectives in social work which are reflected in the debate over anti-racist developments. However, the majority of social workers, given their training, their wider interests in the social world, and the range of pressures they are subject to, would reflect different strands of each of the paradigms discussed above, primarily combining elements of the conservative and the social democratic approaches. As we will see below, in the research interviews, some interviewees drew a distinction between 'traditional' and radical social workers, and by 'traditional' they were referring to a combination of what are here differentiated as conservative and social democratic approaches and concerns. This combination in the 'traditional' approach means that there are often contradictions in the practice of the workers concerned. At certain junctures and in particular contexts, they might operate in a controlling and discriminatory manner, for example pathologising black clients generally, yet on other occasions they might operate in a more anti-discriminatory way, for example in direct work with one of their own black clients.

Black staff and students

One final significant issue relates to the position and treatment of black students and staff within agencies. At the time of CCETSW's developments there was considerable discussion of the effects of institutional racism on these groups. According to Husband (1991), black social workers are likely to experience tension between their personal world and the professional world of social work that is characterised by middle–class norms. Owusu–Bempah (1989) argued:

> Professional training affects the self-concept of students: they designate themselves by an occupational self-reference, as teachers, doctors, nurses, with increasing frequency as they pass through the various stages of professional training. The process also involves internalising social and personality attributes deemed characteristic of the profession one aspires to ... almost every professional training in Britain is tailored to the needs and values of white people; it reflects and reinforces the exclusion of black people from all important spheres of life ... black people are expected to conform to white middle-class needs and values in order to receive a professional service. Those unwilling or unable to do so are therefore pathologised by practitioners such as ... social workers, who are ill-equipped by their eurocentric training to understand or help them. (cited in Clarke, 1993, p 115)

There is a significant pressure on black social workers and students to conform to professional roles in social work agencies. As a result:

> It is not hard for an intellectual or bureaucratised official to convince himself that permutation of and adaptation to the existing power is the smart way to do it ... and it also permits sharing in the perquisites of influence and affluence. (Draper, 1966/97, p 37)

'Professionalism' needs to be recognised as an ideological construct that justifies and reinforces working in ways that reinforce oppression and inequality. Social workers may operate and work in ways that reflects the notion that they are being professional and objective, when in reality they are involved in the "transmission of dominant values and other normative elements of the dominant culture" (Harris, 1991, p 139). This would suggest that black workers can fit into any one of the three 'types' of social worker.

Yet at the same time, black workers and students are likely to experience racism in the workplace and in the myriad aspects of social life, and this would suggest that on the issue of 'race' and racism they are much more likely to express broad social democratic or radical ideas. 'Professionalism' and the experience of institutional racism pull in different directions and represent different pressures on black staff and students. But how they rationalise these pressures will vary according to these workers' wider social work perspectives. Consequently, although racism is an inherent element of the lives of black professionals, their responses to their experiences of racism will be diverse, and will not always be informed by anti-racist analyses. Instead, they will vary from individual to individual and from situation to situation over time. Thus, anti-racism needs to involve white and black workers and should not be seen as the preserve of black workers alone.

Finally, the conceptualisation of three dominant models of social work practice is not static. People's ideas, conceptions and understandings of the world are always subject to change. One way of explaining this is to utilise the concept of 'contradictory consciousness' that was initially developed by the Italian Marxist, Antonio Gramsci. This concept refers to the fact that people, as social agents operating in complex and contradictory class societies, hold a range of potential explanations of the world and of accompanying social relations. The interaction of context and social setting, and the relative strengths and weaknesses of advocates and proponents of various world views, will influence which of these predominates at any given moment. To highlight the concept of contradictory consciousness and how it can operate in practice, it is useful to look at the example of racism and political action in the London docks. In 1968 a section of the London dock labour force reflected their support for Enoch Powell's 'Rivers of Blood' speech by marching to the House of Commons behind banners proclaiming 'Enoch is right'. As a result, the dockers became notorious as a 'racist workforce'. In 1972 the National Front leafleted the docks calling for a march against Asian migrants fleeing oppression in Uganda. The National Front expected the dockers to support their call but the march was a failure and the dock workers took no action. Indeed, in the same year, many of the same dock workers were involved in a major confrontation with the state to release the 'Pentonville Five', five dock shop stewards imprisoned for undertaking unofficial secondary picketing – action which was clearly in support of collectivist notions of trade unionism and solidarity. By 1976 the same dockers went on strike in support of Asian women at the Grunwicks film processing factory, demonstrating elements of a united 'socialist' or collectivist world view, rather than a predominant racist world view. The fact that the same group demonstrated different ideas, values and views at different points of time in relation to different social and political contexts, illustrates that ideas and interpretations of the world are never static, but can alter over time in different contexts. What this example reveals is the dockers' 'contradictory consciousness', which, in 1968 was narrow, racist and divisive, but in 1972 and 1979 more collectivist in nature and form (see Miles and Phizacklea, 1979).

Relating the concept of contradictory consciousness to anti-racist social work requires recognising the range of perspectives and pressures operating within the field – a minority of racists, a minority of anti-racists, a range of managerial pressures, the consequence of economic cuts, various pressures from the 'outside world', and government and media intervention. Each of these is a pressure which will impact on social workers' ideas and perspectives. None of them leads automatically to the conclusion that the anti-racist initiative was doomed to defeat, but it did require an active strategy of engagement to convince the majority of its relevance and importance. As we will see, this was lacking. Instead of argument, education, training and resources, there was policy dictate and imposition. Such a strategy did little to increase the policy's chances of success.

THREE

CCETSW's anti-racist initiative

Social work, as we have noted, is a contradictory practice, and there are a number of perspectives (within the academy and the profession at large) over its appropriate roles, functions and activities. Yet by the late 1980s CCETSW had established a number of clear rules and regulations over the training content and programmes of the new Diploma in Social Work. Central to these developments was the requirement for students to be taught and to be able to facilitate anti-oppressive practice, accompanied by the claim that racism was endemic in British society. As we have noted, this was an important and radical development and it is worth establishing where these ideas developed and why.

A first point to consider is why the anti-racist commitment should have been incorporated within social work education and training at a time when the political climate in Britain was generally hostile to such concerns. This was a period when the Thatcherite project was apparently in full swing (Hall and Jacques, 1983; Gamble, 1988). According to Gamble (1988), part of the Thatcherite political agenda was to establish a new hegemony around a commitment to a free economy and a strong state, and for Hall (1985), central to obtaining such hegemony was the development of an authoritarian populist ideology, within which were implicit references to the 'traditional values' of family, nationhood and 'race'. Thatcherism clearly represented a new political formation, drawing on the tradition of "organic, patriotic Toryism" combined with "a virulent brand of neo-liberal economics and an aggressive religion of the market" (Hall, 1985, p 16), and was a relatively successful attempt to move mainstream political thinking in this direction, shaping a new party political consensus which would seem to be continuing, with some minor countervailing trends, under the present New Labour government (Ludlam and Smith, 1996; Lavalette and Mooney, 1999).

But while 'Thatcherism' may have altered significantly the dominant politics of the main parties in Britain, and sociological and academic discourse over the development of British society in the 1980s, it was never the case that these ideas and values were unproblematically accepted *in toto* by the majority of the population. First, the rhetoric of Thatcherism masked the reality, which often represented a much less dramatic break with economic and social policy than the claims would lead us to believe (Johnson, 1990; Wilson, 1992). Further, as Curran made clear in his critique of Hall's thesis:

> Hall's contention that Thatcherism has undermined 'the popular case for welfare socialism' and 'displaced reformist politics' is contradicted by extensive survey data. A recent survey report [*British Social Attitudes: the 1984 Report* edited by Roger Jowell and Colin Airey] reveals, for example, that the overwhelming majority of people oppose reduced spending on health and education (85%), oppose development of a two-tier health service (64%) and favour a *dirigiste* reformist economic policy – government job creating, construction projects (89%), import controls (72%), price controls (70%), and a government whose first priority is combating unemployment rather than inflation (69%). The same survey reveals, among other things, that Thatcherite talk of incentives has not diminished the view of the great majority (72%), that the gap between high and low incomes is too great. Even those who think that benefits are too high and discourage people from looking for work (35%) are outnumbered by those who think that benefits are too low and cause hardship (46%). (cited in Callinicos, 1985, p 151)

Values and commitments that more recent British Social Attitude reports continue to suggest are deeply embedded in popular consciousness.

As noted already, Gramsci's notion of 'contradictory consciousness' emphasises that social actors can hold a range of apparently conflicting ideas. The experience of social living within capitalist societies promotes competition, conflict and division between social actors, as well as unity, cooperation, mutuality and solidarity. Hence, changes to and within state political culture do not automatically produce changes in people's understanding of the world. Instead, the experiences of life in class-divided societies, and the reality of exploitation and oppression, often sustain oppositional ideas and political practices. This can be seen in the manifestation of opposition to the Thatcherite project which took a number of forms. First, there were, to paraphrase Fox-Piven and Cloward (1977), the 'poor people's movements', the extra-parliamentary struggles such as the inner-city riots (Solomos, 1991; Hussan, 2000), the Great Miners Strike (Callinicos and Simons, 1985), and the Poll Tax Rebellion (Lavalette and Mooney, 1990). Further, despite Thatcher's infamous 'swamping speech', the late 1970s also witnessed confrontations between the National Front and various black organisations, the Anti-

Nazi League and Rock against Racism. These helped to create a climate where racism could be challenged and confronted, and Nazism became 'unacceptable' (Jenkins, forthcoming). It became part of the normal routine of many trade union, community and Left-wing political groups to discuss and confront racism. This is not to suggest that racism vanished – far from it – but the climate was more open to anti-racism than in, for example, France where during the 1980s Le Pen's National Front made significant gains.

A second form of opposition was the growth of the 'reformist left solution' in and around the Labour Party. The early 1980s saw the growth of 'local socialism' (Boddy and Fudge, 1984; Anderson and Cochrane, 1989), when a number of Left-wing Labour councils attempted to use their local base to promote alternative, non-market-based political solutions to local problems (Lavalette and Mooney, 2000). At the same time, the growth of Women's and Black Sections in the Labour Party represented an important development within the Labour Party and again, within local government (Bruegel and Kean, 1995). In some senses these developments represented conflict over strategy within the New Social Movements. During the 1960s such groups had been much more concerned with politics outside parliament and the development of alternatives to mainstream politics. During the 1980s, however, the growth of Women's and Black Sections represented both an acknowledgement of issues of gender and 'race' inequality by the Labour Party, and an accommodation with the Labour Party by a number of activists from these movements (see Lavalette, 1999). This led to a situation where issues of gender and racism became more visible in Labour Party discussions and documentation, and where Labour-controlled councils increasingly adopted Equal Opportunities statements, although there were regional variations in the commitment of local authorities to implementing anti-discriminatory policies, which, in turn, impacted on the development of anti-racist practices and procedures. For example, much more progressive initiatives took place in areas such as inner London where, in the early 1980s, radical equal opportunities programmes were pioneered by authorities such as Lambeth and the then Greater London Council, rather than in areas such as Lancashire.

These developments coincided with the growth and expansion of the 'race relations industry' (Sivanandan, 1991), and led to a situation where, despite the ascendancy of the Conservative Party under Margaret Thatcher, there was a developing political culture within the Labour Party, local government and the equal opportunities community that stressed the racist nature of British society. Finally, changes within social work, the expansion of social work services, the impact of radical social work perspectives on social work activity, and the role of some academics, put pressure on CCETSW to recognise various forms of oppression. These three elements – popular opposition to some elements of Thatcherism, the legislative agenda of municipal socialism, and pressures from sections of the profession – produced a culture which was to be influential within and on CCETSW. But a final crucial element in the emergence of the anti-racist programme was the struggle of the black community itself.

The emergence of anti-racist social work initiatives during the 1980s and early 1990s was a direct consequence of black struggle and resistance, and a developing critique of social work and social work education from an anti-racist perspective. Many black students and social workers had struggled for years to challenge the failure of social work courses to address anti-racism effectively, and had been among the main catalysts in stimulating change. The interventions of black social work practitioners can be analysed in the context of the long experience of anti-racist struggles within Britain's black communities and a history of white and black cooperation over anti-racist political initiatives (Heinemann, 1972; Ben-Tovim et al, 1986; Wadsworth, 1998).

In the 1940s and 1950s Britain was a hostile, unwelcoming environment steeped in the ideology of racial superiority, and black organisations were formed around the need to protect black communities (Miles and Phizacklea, 1984). During the early 1960s a variety of black organisations were set up to organise against both discriminatory legislation and racist practices, and during the 1970s their numbers increased. They were influential in exposing the persistence of racism in society and the discriminatory practices that the black community were facing at the hands of the British state, particularly the racism which black youth were facing at the hands of the police and the courts (Denney, 1983; Gilroy, 1987; NACRO, 1993). They were also influential in resisting discriminatory and negative social welfare developments. For example, during the 1970s and 1980s, black women in particular were involved in tenants and squatters campaigns, and in struggles against the abuses of the education system (Bryan et al, 1985). The black press, for example *The Voice*, was also influential in the 1980s in documenting the social and economic deprivation and discrimination faced by black families. At the same time, various locally based monitoring groups were set up to record incidents of racist violence and establish structures of resistance within the black communities.

The resistance to discriminatory welfare legislation has also manifested itself in the social work arena, where black organisations and black practitioners have, over the years, been increasingly critical of the nature of social services provision for the black community. This has been the result of increasing concern that "patterns of discrimination and disadvantage seem to be reproduced and reinforced within the operations of social work, rather than being compensated for by its provision" (Ely and Denney, 1987, p 99). During the 1970s black social workers began questioning the content of social work and its relevance to the black community. This was starkly revealed by the under-representation of black clients in the caring and preventive elements of social work provision (Bryan et al, 1985; Duncan, 1986; Ahmad, 1990), and their over-representation in its controlling elements (Ahmad, 1990; Thompson, 1993). Black people's behaviour and family life were evidently judged particularly harshly by social work professionals, especially in terms of mental health and childcare, revealing that black parents are more likely to have their children removed and placed in residential and foster care (Bebbington and Miles, 1989), and to receive more severe diagnoses of mental illness and confinement under the Mental Health Act (Francis, 1991).

Black social workers and black voluntary groups have, over the years, fought to expose the fact that these disturbing trends are a consequence of unacknowledged and unintentional racism based on negative stereotypes and assumptions of black groups. For example, Afro-Caribbean families are often pathologised, with mothers seen as being too strong, whereas an Asian family is seen as problematic because the mother's position is considered weak and uninfluential (Skellington and Morris, 1992). Black groups have been instrumental in exposing the destructive effects of these incorrect and negative interpretations of black behaviour and family structures in areas such as child protection (CCCS, 1982; Roys, 1988), and in highlighting the need to confront the ethnocentricity that informs the professional judgement of social workers (Arnold and James, 1988). They have also demonstrated the negative effects for the black community of stereotypes expressed in positive terms, such as 'Asians look after their own' (Cadman and Chakrabarti, 1991). As a result, the black community itself has done much of the work to make social services more accessible and appropriate to the needs of the black community.

This has been particularly pertinent in relation to adoption and fostering. In the 1960s concern was beginning to be expressed regarding the problem posed for social workers by the significant numbers of black and mixed parentage children in care (Denney, 1983), and during the 1970s significant sections of the black community, angry at the pathologisation of family relationships, methods of childcare, and the number of black children in care, began to organise to counter such negative perceptions. They instigated developments such as the 'Soul Kids Campaign', which was the first concerted attempt at black family recruitment in Britain, planned and coordinated by a group of London-based social workers. In 1980 the new Black Families Unit was set up by the London Borough of Lambeth and the Independent Adoption Society to recruit, assess and approve black people as foster and adoptive parents for black children, and in 1982 the Association of Black Social Workers and Allied Professionals was formed, which made transracial adoption its major concern (Bryan et al,1985; Coombe and Little, 1986). These developments were attempts to counter the assumption that black families willing to foster or adopt were almost non-existent. They were also a response to the failure in social work to recognise the alienation of black children in white care settings, and acted as a challenge to definitions of normality being imposed on black families by white practitioners. These challenges to the discriminatory and ethnocentric nature of social work provision fitted significantly and decisively into social work education and training during the 1980s and 1990s.

Within social work, it was during the 1980s that assimilationist/integrationist and multicultural theories came under attack, and racism became increasingly perceived as a fundamental institutional problem structuring social work policies and practices (Husband, 1991). Many black activists were challenging theories based on crude cultural stereotypes which reinforced notions of cultural pathology, strengthened ideas of white cultural superiority and obscured the material conditions of black people in society (Ahmed, 1991). They were also criticising initiatives, such as Racial Awareness Training, for their emphasis on the personal and individual manifestation of racism (Sivanandan, 1985). These debates all contributed to the development of anti-racist social work education and training that would be "informed by the practical issues that affect the [black] community in society" (Francis, 1991, p 184). They were challenges that indicated a more systematic and determined attempt to introduce specific anti-racist requirements into social work education and training, and signified a fundamental shift in the anti-discriminatory theoretical perspectives that had influenced social work practice over the years.

A further specific pressure to address racism in social work education came from black social work organisations such as the Mickleton Group. In the late 1980s they held a number of 'alternative conferences' that again criticised the eurocentric and middle-class nature of social work education, and directly led to the creation by CCETSW of a Black Perspectives Committee (Strong, 1995).

The combined effect of these various factors and concerns was to persuade CCETSW of the importance of tackling the issue of 'race' and racism within social work education and training, and this explains why, despite a political climate apparently hostile to progressive politics, CCETSW could make a commitment to an anti-racist social work programme.

CCETSW's anti-racist agenda

In the late 1980s and early 1990s CCETSW responded to these criticisms of social work education and training in a number of ways that demonstrated a serious and radical commitment to look at routes to anti-racist social work practice. CCETSW began to question seriously why social work practice was so deficient in anti-racist initiatives.

In November 1988 CCETSW formally adopted an anti-racist policy that stated:

> CCETSW believes that racism is endemic in the values, attitudes and structures of British society including that of social services and social work education. CCETSW recognises that the effects of racism on black people are incompatible with the values of social work and therefore seeks to combat racist practices in all areas of its responsibilities. (CCETSW, 1991b, p 6)

As a result the Diploma in Social Work (Paper 30) further stipulated learning requirements in relation to anti-racist social work, which included:

> Recognising the implications of political, economic, racial, social and cultural factors upon service delivery, financing services and resource analysis;

> Demonstrating an awareness of both individual and institutional racism and ways to combat both through anti-racist practice;

> Developing an awareness of the inter-relationships of the processes of structural oppression, race, class and gender and

> Working in an ethnically sensitive way. (CCETSW, 1989a, pp 15, 16, 19)

CCETSW was clearly committed to training social workers to recognise the nature of structural racism and to facilitate anti-racist practice. The intention was to create a new workforce of anti-racist social workers. But it was not just trainees who were to reflect these values. Paper 30 included compulsory requirements for programmes leading to the Diploma in Social Work. Programme providers must, for example, develop:

> ... clear and explicit anti-discrimination and anti-racist policies, and explicit practices and procedures which provide evidence that these policies will be implemented and monitored in all aspects of the programme. (CCETSW, 1989a, p 22)

The programme providers, the colleges, universities and the placement agencies, were expected to implement and *monitor* anti-racist policies and practices.

CCETSW also recognised the importance of practice teachers within the profession, and their key training role with student social workers. Paper 26.3 (CCETSW, 1989b), which governed the Council's approval of agencies for practice learning and its requirements for the accreditation and training of practice teachers, was an integral part of its commitment to improve the quality of placements for students. This paper gave practice teachers and their employing institutions a key role in enabling students to undertake anti-racist and anti-discriminatory social work. Practice teachers were required to link theory and practice in the area of anti-oppressive social work practice, and were charged with keeping up to date with the current debates in this area. CCETSW's approval of agencies for practice learning insisted on the provision of high quality learning opportunities within an environment that required anti-discriminatory practice.

Finally, in 1988, to underpin these developments, CCETSW launched its five year Curriculum Development Project, which included meetings with black students and an all-black conference of students and workers from the North of England. This project was 'grass-roots led' and "guided by the understanding that racism is a structural phenomenon whose elimination requires a strong anti-racist ideological commitment" (Patel, 1991, p 11). Anti-racist training materials were produced and published, created by the joint work of students, practitioners, tutors and researchers using a wide pool of knowledge and skills. These included training packs on children and families, elders, mental health, learning difficulties, probation and practice teaching. This substantial publishing effort was an important contribution to CCETSW's anti-racist requirements, and was also a valuable resource for the many practice teachers and tutors who were concerned about their lack of knowledge and awareness regarding anti-racist issues, and expressing a demand for relevant published material (Patel, 1991).

These developments all constituted a fundamental attempt by CCETSW to make anti-racism a central requirement of social work training, and a central component of good social work practice. The programme requirements were clear. In order to activate anti-racist practice, at least three conditions had to be met:

- Students needed to develop the appropriate knowledge and skills to implement anti-racist practice;
- Programme providers (higher education institutions and social work agencies) had to have clear anti-racist policies which should be appropriately monitored, and be committed to developing anti-racist practice;
- Practice teachers should be adequately trained and prepared to facilitate anti-racist education and training.

These were the three central elements of CCETSW's strategy to establish anti-racist social work. The extent to which these stated aims were implemented, and the range of barriers that students faced, forms the basis of the research findings presented in the next three chapters.

FOUR

Research findings and the implementation of Paper 30

In 1990 and 1991, at the time that CCETSW was introducing Paper 30, a research project was set up at the University of Central Lancashire to investigate its implementation. The research was based on in-depth semi-structured interviews with black and white students from the first two cohort years of the Diploma in Social Work, and with their respective practice teachers. Each student was interviewed three times while they were on placement, in order to ascertain if, over a period of two years, the developments were having an impact on education, training and practice within agencies.

As we have noted, the rules and regulations for the Diploma in Social Work required practice teachers and the institutions in which they were located to enable students (both black and white) to effectively carry out anti-racist practice. The process of implementing the research immediately confirmed the nature of institutional racism in social work agencies, identified as the systematic outcome of institutional systems and routine practices which, in effect, discriminate against members of ethnic minority populations (Williams, 1985; Husband, 1991). As Husband has noted, this can lead:

> ... to the unhappy consequence that nice people can be accused of being culpable of participating in generating racist outcomes [and that] it is very disquieting for anyone to be told that independently of their own sense of personal agency they are perpetuating a form of racist practice. (Husband, 1991, p 53)

The research revealed three institutional indicators as being instrumental in reinforcing and reproducing racism in social work agencies: the representation of black clients within agencies, the representation of black staff, and the effectiveness of anti-discriminatory policies.

Black client representation

Social work clients have historically, tended to come from the most disadvantaged and socially deprived areas (Barclay Report, 1982; Clarke, 1993; Jones, 1998). This research was carried out in Lancashire, a county faced with disproportionate levels of poverty, poor housing, poor health and education, particularly among its black community (Lancashire County Council Planning Department, 1986; Blackburn Borough Council, 1996), which would indicate a real need for assistance from the personal social services. Yet findings from the research pointed to the under-representation of black clients in most aspects of provision, and the inadequacy of resources to develop anti-discriminatory practice. By the early 1990s the culture and reality of cuts and budget restrictions had been in place since the mid-1970s (Langan, 1993), and this was clearly affecting existing services. The Commission for Racial Equality highlighted the consequences in 1989, when they suggested that although social work has legal duties to ensure that black groups receive equal and appropriate services, social services departments were not implementing legislative requirements enshrined in the 1976 Race Relations Act.

From the interviews black students suggested that there were a range of barriers that affected black clients seeking help and assistance from social services departments. The students' concerns reflected a number of themes. First, several students highlighted the problem of stereotyping:

> "White social workers are not used to seeing black faces in social services departments and they do not like it. They still assume Asian families can take care of all their own problems."

> "One student brought a video in which showed situations with clients and one of the clients was a young Asian woman who was sat there clearly upset. I was fascinated by the replies [from other staff] and amazed that everyone's first thought was that she couldn't speak English, which had never crossed my mind. Surely black people have been in this country long enough for people not to be automatically thinking along these lines. They couldn't see why I was annoyed."

> "I did ask questions about black clients and they said that they had an Asian elderly client ... *and didn't really have any problems with him at all* [author's emphasis]. I also asked about black clients at the hospital

and they said that as soon as they leave hospital they just go back to their families. Obviously it is their assumption that they have a family to go back to. Even at the day care centre I asked if they had any black clients and they said no. When I asked if they knew why they just said 'Oh, I think they have a centre of their own'."

These accounts reveal the continuing hold of a range of cultural stereotypes within social work departments, and how they are translated into practice. In this respect, the focus on 'assumed cultural practices' detracts from any awareness of or attempt to deal with institutional racism.

A second set of concerns raised by students related to resource provision for the black community:

"There is nothing here and I have come to believe that the needs of ethnic minorities will never be met. I sincerely believe that we need to develop almost parallel services run privately by agencies. It is against my principles but I cannot see any other way of meeting needs. We need resources, experience and theoretical knowledge of their needs. It goes back to awareness regarding injustices in society and being sensitive to the needs and problems of those who are discriminated against."

"I asked how social services assist the black community and my practice teacher said that they just pay lip-service and that nothing concrete gets done. They only have one section 11 worker here, and they think it is enough in this big team."

"There are no resources here but I would know where to go within the black community. That is based on my own personal knowledge but I don't think white social workers would be aware of it. They would probably say 'sorry, we haven't got the resources'."

In an era of financial cuts, providing resources for all clients is deeply problematic. In this context, establishing services for the black community (even basic provision) comes up against financial restraint in local government and social work agencies. In this sense, basic needs are not being met due to resources concerns. In these circumstances provision for the black community often rests on the individual knowledge of social workers and the black voluntary sector, in a way that is far more extensive than it would be for white clients.

Notwithstanding this, some students noted that practitioners contrasted the 'lack of resources' available to all clients with 'the special treatment' they thought minority ethnic communities received:

> "I think that the general policy at the moment is that we have not got resources for the indigenous population so why should ethnic minorities have resources?"

There was also a lack of awareness from within the minority ethnic communities about the role of social workers (in part reflecting the social work department's non-involvement with the black community):

> "You have a credibility problem. In the indigenous population people have heard of social workers or let's say they have a rough idea of what they do. The Asian population doesn't have a clue. Do social workers help or do they have power [ie referring to the controlling role of social work]?"

However, some students reported more disturbing 'race-blind' or racist attitudes:

> "To staff here culture and 'race' don't matter. You treat all people the same and because they have no black clients here they say they have no problem."

> "My practice teacher asked me what I would think about them [a children's agency] having a golliwog. I said that I would find it offensive because of the connotations that it carries, and how it is perceived. But she had no idea."

Finally, a number of students thought that raising issues of black client representation and the needs of the black community was unwelcome within agencies. Several thought that by raising the issues they were somehow identified as 'troublemakers', and as one said:

> "I think one of our roles which is important is that we don't upset the balance and don't appear threatening in any way."

Some black students also came into contact with racism outside social work agencies, particularly from the general public and other state professionals. For example, one student said:

"I have a client who is mentally ill who was sleeping on the streets, but he has now been given a furnished flat as I got him a community care grant. But there have been problems with the neighbours complaining about his behaviour as sometimes he howls like a dog. The neighbours have said things like his behaviour must be 'in his breeding'."

Another student became involved in a case regarding immigration, which exposed the discriminatory nature of legislation:

"I got a case to work with a Bangladeshi chap who doesn't speak English or my language, and I was horrified when I read his file. He has had an incredible raw deal and is in a psychiatric ward, which you can understand if you know his circumstances. He arrived in Britain in 1957 and got a passport, and in 1972 he applied for his family to join him. They have not joined him yet and he is now 65, which is old by Asian standards. He hasn't been able to get his family over for the ludicrous reason that he was inconsistent during an interview. I mean, how do you expect a person who doesn't speak English and is depressed and agitated to be consistent. Because he was uncooperative, he was accused of trying to 'pull the wool over their eyes'. I felt so angry that I decided to write a letter to the Home Office and my practice teacher agreed. In my last office they would not have allowed me to write such a letter, but until this is dealt with we are not going to be able to help him."

The accounts of black students revealed how racism manifests itself in the institutional practices and procedures of social work agencies. First, in the application of unhelpful, inaccurate and obsolete cultural stereotypes of the black population; second, in the lack of knowledge and awareness among white social workers which has a negative impact on service provision; and third, in racist stereotypes evident in the wider community. There were also instances when black students were confronted with the structural impact of racism on their clients' lives. Further, most black students at some point in their placement questioned the nature of black client representation and resources available for the black community.

But the level of concern and awareness around issues of racism among black students varied. This appeared to be related to both the level of professional experience that individual students possessed, and their general social work perspectives. For example, those students relatively 'new' to social work, whose expectations were shaped by the anti-racist teaching programme on the social work course, tended to be more shocked at the racism which they witnessed or experienced within agencies. In this context, students with little social work experience appeared to have expectations that agencies would somehow reflect the same anti-racist concerns, and of course this was CCETSW's intention. But clearly there was a tension between the theory and practice of social work education and training. In contrast, more experienced black students, although concerned regarding the treatment of black clients, were not surprised at their status within social work agencies and the lack of resources. Their own experiences had 'prepared' them for the fact that issues of racism were unlikely to be prioritised in the field. But, it is equally important to stress that all black students do not share the same perspectives over issues of discrimination, inequality and anti-oppressive practice. Some black students looked towards familial and community support networks, others looked towards social work as an agency to improve the lives, however marginally, of all the oppressed, while others looked on their role as being advocates of the dispossessed against the structural inequities of society. Black students, like their white counterparts, had a range of political perspectives and attitudes, and this in part affected the degree to which they felt confident to tackle or raise issues of racism. Several students also voiced their concern that raising such issues could damage either the successful completion of placements or future job prospects so, as such, it was easier and less threatening to compromise, and identify with, rather than challenge, dominant institutional values.

The accounts of white students revealed that it was students who could be described as 'radical' in their approach to social work practice and their understanding of racism in society who were most aware and concerned about the status of black clients and the discrimination that they faced in social work agencies. They were also committed to developing anti-racist practice. In contrast, more conservative white students tended to ignore or dismiss the importance of such questions or look to black social workers to have the solution. However, the majority of white students, although not hostile to anti-racist developments, did not appear confident in discussing or dealing with them while on placement. For example, one student stated:

> "I have one black client who is moving from residential care to the community, and he experiences a lot of discrimination because of his disability and because he is black. I have been trying to get an

Asian group involved as he has lost contact with the Asian community, but initially I did not know who to approach, and I didn't want to offend the black worker here, and I felt terrible that I had to go to a black worker to find out about resources, because they don't come to us about resources for white clients. I had heard that in the Asian community the mentally ill are rejected but it is not something I have come across."

Questions regarding black client representation revealed that, generally, the lack of an institutional response to racism leads at best to individual endeavours to provide a positive service for black clients (which may or may not be based on a series of unchallenged stereotypes), and, at worst, no attempt at all. In all instances, however, among both black and white students, those who were able to incorporate discussions regarding 'race' and racism in the most constructive and worthwhile manner were students with radical practice teachers. For example, the black student who wrote to the Home Office regarding his client stated that:

"I consider my practice teacher a 'radical' social worker. More 'traditional' social workers would not have been as moved and concerned. 'Traditional' social workers do not have a commitment to social injustice, which I feel is an important part of our work."

Although students with social democratic practice teachers initially felt able to address anti-racist issues, a lack of knowledge and awareness and/or a degree of defensiveness among practice teachers usually meant that the issues were not dealt with in an informative or constructive manner. As a result, students eventually began to avoid the subject. The students who fared worst were those with conservative practice teachers, who, in several cases, refused to take anti-discriminatory debates on board and were outwardly hostile to the issues (something I will refer to later).

Black staff representation

All practice teachers participating in the research project were white, and there did not appear to be any black practice teachers in any of the agencies that were involved in the research. Such a situation was not unusual. Williams (1985) believed it strange that there was a shortage of black practice teachers when, for a decade or more, black students had been qualifying for social work courses, while Stokes (1996) indicated that although many black workers were interested in becoming practice teachers, few were encouraged and supported to do so. Social work academics such as Husband have also voiced their concern that:

> The marginal location of black workers within social work institutions is itself an important factor in facilitating a dominant white definition of 'professionalism'. Professional ideologies generate artificial boundaries of competence and responsibility which define correct procedures and acceptable targets for 'professional' intervention. (Husband, 1991, p 55)

As well as being aware of the under-representation of black clients within social work agencies, black students were also concerned about the under-representation and marginalisation of black staff. As one student said:

> "There is one Section 11 worker here and the department view is that he should go out into the community. But there are thousands of Asians and one man cannot do the job. For example, there are schools here that are 75% Asian and there are Asian cases going through the courts."

There was also some evidence of Section 11 workers being treated differently:

> "I have worked in social work agencies where qualified workers look down on Section 11 workers."

Black students also spoke of the hostility of some white staff when black staff and students were given access to professional training (part of the attempt to increase black worker representation):

> "There are social work assistants who have tried to get on CQSW courses and have failed because there is so much competition. Then when they see a black worker accepted, they resent it."

However, again, in relation to their past experiences, there were mixed responses to the suggestion that social work agencies would benefit from employing more black staff. Black students who were relatively new to social work tended to express the view that this would be a positive development:

"It would help to have more black staff. For example, where I am working, there are no black care assistants, and it would have been interesting to see if they would be more aware of the needs of Asian clients."

"It would be a positive thing at all levels. It is now something that I worry about."

Experienced black students, however, were more cautious:

"It would help to have more black staff but they would have to be the right sort of black worker, in the way that good black workers can give off positive images and get cooperation and service provision, then a bad black worker can take it all away again. If you have a 'bull in a china shop' approach on 'race' then you get people's backs up and they 'put up the shutters' even more than they do now."

"I don't think that more black staff would make a difference, and just because I am Asian it doesn't mean that I am tuned in with anti-discriminatory policies."

In this respect, more experienced black students were concerned that black staff should demonstrate competence without upsetting or antagonising other members of staff, and should tread carefully when discussing issues associated with 'race' and racism. These concerns reflect the difficulties associated with imposing an initiative in a less than receptive environment, and are also suggestive of the 'pressures' on social workers to conform to the dominant 'professional' ethos within agencies. There was also a concern among more experienced workers, that less experienced black students might negatively reflect on their own abilities. There was disquiet that black students might be perceived as being knowledgeable about aspects of anti-racist practice, solely by virtue of being black.

Although in most agencies black staff were under-represented, there were exceptions that emphasised, that with commitment from the agency and appropriate resources being made available, it was possible to begin promoting an anti-racist professional culture. One student spoke of the benefits of being placed in an agency that did employ black staff:

"There are four black staff here and they are all social workers. I am in contact with other offices that have black staff, even some in

> management. I have joined a 'Black Women in Local Authority' group and there is also a 'Black in Care' group. I find it quite enlightening and wonderful.... There is support and a sharing of problems.... I went to see a fostering officer who is a black woman and in her office there were pictures of her family and of Jamaica which I have never come across before.... It is nice for people to realise that you exist and that you can contribute to society in a positive way, rather than a negative way all the time."

In this example, the agency was also committed to dealing with all aspects of racism, and supporting black staff, which did represent an attempt to tackle institutional racism – this example is a crucially important one, as it emphasises that things can be done to counter institutional racism within social work agencies.

Again, it was more radical white students who demonstrated an awareness and concern regarding the status of black social work staff. For example, one student stated that she wanted to incorporate an analysis based on anti-racism into her placement report, but was unable to do so because of an absence of black clients and the attitude of her practice teacher who was overtly hostile to such a suggestion. She stated:

> "In my initial interview I asked about black clients and Section 11 workers, but they have no Section 11 workers here, and my practice teacher doesn't seem interested. I was a bit dubious because one of my objectives is to explore how they use Section 11 money. It wasn't so much that they have not got Section 11 workers, but that they don't see it as important.... At the moment all they do here is complain about anti-discriminatory attitudes and practices."

The accounts of black students demonstrated that the marginalisation of black workers is an important factor in facilitating a dominant white definition of professionalism, and that the pressure to conform was exacerbated when students did not have the support of other black staff, or white workers sympathetic to anti-discriminatory initiatives. Again, while on placement, it was students with radical practice teachers who were more able to discuss black staff representation in an open and honest manner. However, more experienced black students fared better, due to their familiarity with institutional norms and the development of a range of coping mechanisms.

Anti-racist policies

The existence of anti-discriminatory policies and the seriousness afforded them, a commitment to providing resources and provision of ongoing education can all impact on the culture of an organisation, and influence the attitudes, awareness, and commitment of staff to anti-discriminatory practice. This in turn can affect the level of discrimination that black staff experience in social work agencies and how racist incidents are dealt with.

The 1976 Race Relations Act had (and continues to have) relevance for anti-racist social work provision. It provided the legal basis for local authorities to provide appropriate services for the black community, and stipulated that action could be taken against employers for both direct and indirect discrimination. Section 71 of the Act stated that local authorities need to:

> Make appropriate arrangements with a view to securing that their various functions are carried out with due regard to the need to eliminate unlawful discrimination and to promote equality of opportunity and good relations between different racial groups.

Social work departments are also covered by Section 20 of the Act that outlaws discrimination in the provision of services "by deliberately omitting to provide them, or as regards their quality or the manner or the terms on which they are provided".

CCETSW's anti-racist policy and its requirements for the Diploma in Social Work and the Accreditation of Practice Teachers also recognises the need to address racism in social work, and incorporate methods and requirements to facilitate this. However, in spite of such policies and recommendations, Social Services Inspectorate research (1987) found an almost total failure to formulate effective policies. They also came to the conclusion that implementation and monitoring were not in evidence.

Students' comments while they were on placement reflected these concerns, as most were either unaware or only vaguely aware of anti-discriminatory legislation, and there was no evidence that they were incorporated into the learning agenda in an influential or useful manner, despite the fact that several students did attempt to discuss them.

First, a number of students noted that while there *may* have been formal policies, these were not embedded in daily practice or were not part of the local agency culture:

"I talked to the Director of Social Services who gave me feedback on policies, and he said that where discrimination is concerned they do have policies and they go on Racial Awareness Training courses.... But if I was discriminated against I don't think I would know what to do."

"In terms of equal opportunities policies, there is one somewhere at headquarters, but staff are not aware of it. I have asked to look at them, but they don't know where to get them from and they are not actually being implemented."

"I did ask about policies when the placement started but no one seemed to have any information. There is a lot of talk about equal opportunities policies but very little in practice."

"They have things on paper but it doesn't mean they take things seriously."

"I do know that policies exist, and there are a lot concerned with childcare and mental health, but there is very little on anti-racist policies.... Some social workers ... have to face the fact that black clients have needs, and policies are also needed to highlight the implications of being racist."

The implementation of equal opportunities policies is something to be welcomed. But these examples all emphasise the danger of policy merely becoming an abstract blueprint that fails to have any connection to daily practices within organisations, or that fails to alter the working culture in any way. Merely passing policy at local government or institutional level is not the same as implementing or developing policy, both of which require commitment and resources within institutions.

Other students reported working in agencies where the issue was simply ignored:

"There are no anti-racist policies here. You see it is all based on Christian values, and I was told that it did not matter that there were no policies, because they do not have any black clients."

"I have worked in places where it comes down to the attitudes of workers who will ignore policies.... I know that they are not worth the paper they are written on."

"I think they fall back on their religious faith for policy … it seems to be understood that you treat people as equally as you can."

Some white students were also critical regarding the effectiveness of anti-discriminatory policies. One white student who was particularly keen to develop anti-racist practice described how her practice teacher responded:

"I have asked my practice teacher about policies relating to clients. His response was that he is not aware of anything but there should be something about. I pushed it further … and he eventually rang for information, but he said 'I have got this stroppy student who is insisting I ring'…. There are no clear policies in this agency…. I spent a morning at the Equal Opportunities Unit in the next large town team, and they have very good policy statements which they are actually implementing. However, they said it takes a long time, as their statement was written five years ago and they are still plugging away at it. It was quite a relief to find that there are people interested in doing things. My practice teacher knows policies in terms of interviewing but he thinks they are a 'pain in the neck'. He may not want to stick to them but he knows he has to. The staff here said that it took them a while to get him to stop being racist in terms of his language, and he is more careful now."

The accounts of black and white students demonstrated that although many were aware of the potential of anti-discriminatory policies, they rarely found them introduced or implemented in a constructive and meaningful manner, and were sceptical about their effectiveness. They also recognised that policy statements by themselves do not automatically eliminate discrimination in institutions, and were concerned that in practice, policies could be used to cover up inaction or indifference.

The situation was made worse for students placed with conservative practice teachers, as they tended to be hostile to legislative developments associated with addressing inequalities in society. In these cases, students, depending on their confidence and ability, were left to pursue such issues alone, but as the Social Services Inspectorate (1987) revealed, without the active support of their agencies, individuals can only make a marginal impact on the nature of service provision.

Part of CCETSW's anti-racist initiative was that placement providers were *required* to provide students with an environment conducive to facilitating appropriate anti-racist social work practice. However, the research revealed that, in many cases, this was difficult or impossible, due to the institutional nature of racism within social work agencies, and, in some cases, the hostile attitude of individual practice teachers. This resulted in discrimination and the de-prioritisation of the needs of black communities, and superficial 'race-related' work when anti-racism was reduced to cultural activities, or a minor standing item at the end of a team meeting. Work with black clients was often left to Section 11 workers, but this often led to the marginalisation of black workers, who were often perceived as *the* workers for all black clients. Thus, while Section 11 funding was important in establishing services for the black community, it also had the consequence of de-prioritising the needs of black clients and black workers in terms of mainstream social work practice. This is a prime example of a welfare activity being contradictory in its impact, bringing both 'benefits' and 'costs' to workers and users.

Further interviews with students revealed that in an atmosphere of financial cuts, and increasing stress and competition for promotion and training places, the *abstract* imposition of anti-oppressive policies could lead to resentment and bitterness from white workers at particular junctures. For example, black students and workers are devalued, and are often assumed to have got a job or a student place because of the colour of their skin, and the fact of black under-representation does not undermine the racist stereotype. This is important. It emphasises that, in a structurally racist society with a dominant racist culture, a lack of resources and the pressures arising from increasing workloads, can all mesh with racist stereotyping and racist myths to provoke hostility and racism. Miles and Phizacklea have argued that:

> It is ... immediate daily experience which leads a substantial proportion of white workers to have such firmly held negative views of black workers, in this context of a national culture which is itself racist. (1979, p 120)

This is not to justify racism, but to emphasise the material circumstances which promote racist divisions, and to suggest that material realities exist within social work agencies as much as they do in the 'outside world'. Of course, other 'solutions' and explanations can be offered to account for the pressure of cuts and workloads, but this requires the intervention of activists willing to challenge racism and offer collectivist alternatives to the problems of both social workers and their clients.

Yet, in this bleak picture, there were also positive insights in workplaces with black support groups and committed anti-racist social workers, where anti-discriminatory policies can be more fully operated precisely because they are not abstract top-down impositions, but are an integral part of the work culture of agencies. The experiences of one or two students emphasised that anti-racist social work practice can operate and function as part of the 'routine' of social work agencies when there are both clear and known anti-racist policies, and committed anti-racist social work activists. There was also evidence that debates regarding 'race', racism and anti-racist practice that took place within the university before placements began, raised 'theoretical' concerns which led a number of students to challenge agency 'norms'. They also made it less likely that students would operate, unconsciously or perhaps unwillingly, in a discriminatory manner. This was a vital finding, given the moves towards competency-based learning for social work education and training.

Finally, many students seemed to hold a 'contradictory consciousness' with regard to anti-racist practice. White students often worked 'unknowingly' or 'unquestioningly' in agencies with little concern for issues of anti-racism, but faced with the needs of black clients, or university assessment requirements, they focused, often critically, on the lack of facilities or policies. These students were not racists, but at times they worked in ways that reflected and incorporated the institutional racism of social work agencies. Black students were under pressure to appear 'professional' and to accept agency procedures and practices, but at the same time, were acutely aware of the negative consequences this had for black workers and clients. However, again, in the right environment, with a committed practice teacher, support groups, and a general culture and atmosphere of anti-racism, students were able to explore and participate in anti-racist practice in a much more positive manner.

Dealing with racism

As a result of the nature of racism within social work agencies, the failure to implement anti-discriminatory policies, and the lack of awareness and/or hostility of many practice teachers regarding racism and anti-racist strategies, it is not surprising that for black students, dealing with the racism that they experienced while on placement was extremely difficult. It also created problems for white students who wished to incorporate anti-discriminatory practice into their learning experience.

Throughout their placements most black students remained fearful of the consequences of discussing racist incidents, as they felt it might jeopardise their relationships with other staff and affect the successful completion of their placement. This was made more difficult, as much of the racism which they experienced in agencies came from social work staff and other welfare professionals. In a few instances this led to a situation where the staff that black students looked to for support were often the same staff that were exhibiting direct and indirect racist attitudes. However, the accounts below reveal that, despite their fears and the lack of support and awareness in agencies, many black students did attempt to challenge racism using strategies ranging from confrontation to 'education'.

Black students' responses revealed that it was the most experienced students who had worked within white statutory agencies, and/or students with a particularly strong commitment to anti-racism, who were most confident in dealing with racism. The accounts that follow demonstrate how racism manifested itself within agencies, and how black students attempted to deal with it:

"If someone makes racist remarks to me I will certainly deal with it myself. But I am quite a strong person, whereas some black students would be scared to deal with it.... However, I do think that it could threaten my placement success, and if an experienced black social worker started challenging the ways of working here, his progress would be seriously undermined. But if he remained quiet about such issues perhaps his promotion chances would be greater."

"One day I was parking my car and the attendant said 'Can I help you?' and then asked what I was doing. A few weeks later another car park attendant asked me exactly the same thing. I think there is an assumption that black people do not belong here...."

"There is another [white] second year student here, and she doesn't speak to me or acknowledge me, and she has told other social workers that black workers find it much easier than white workers to get on courses, and that they are not as able as white students."

"The senior [social worker] is clearly racist, but placements are vital to passing your course, and I don't know what would happen if I challenged him."

"I think we all have difficulty dealing with racism on placement.... I mean social workers do make racist comments, which creates a tension that is not easy to tackle.... I tackle it [racism] by educating people and mean that in the sincerest sense. I put people down if they make comments I find hard to accept, and I try to demean them. If they are humiliated, they take a different stance which allows me to go in and talk about things.... I had a problem with a particular work colleague.... One day when we were really short-staffed we had to close the duty desk for two hours, and an Asian bloke who didn't know this, and who had come several miles without a car didn't know this, so I decided to let him in. My [white] colleague then walked in and was really rude, ignorant and obnoxious. He had this mythical faith in the British 'race' which was obvious from conversations with him. He told my client in a rude way to 'go home', and I blew my top, which led to a confrontation. I told him that I was sick of his petty comments regarding black people. It was the turning point for him, and now he asks some really soul-searching questions which he would never have asked me before."

The student, in this case, appears to believe that confrontation is the only way of challenging racist individuals, although his account reveals that this is usually the result of a series of direct and indirect racist outbursts. Confrontation, therefore, is not the initial response, but the consequence of a history of racist ideas, attitudes and practices going unchallenged in the workplace.

Other black workers made attempts to counter the stereotypical assumptions within agencies:

"The clerical assistant here is nice and friendly, but when we were talking about my life she was obviously thinking in terms of cultural stereotypes such as arranged marriages, and she asked me if I used to live in a mud hut. I had to start explaining things to her, but I think I will have to bring in some videos or books and show her what the situation really is. You see, like other social work staff, she is reflecting all the stereotypical images she reads and hears about."

Another student stated that:

"I am always willing to sit down and talk to people about things. I discussed things with staff like I prefer to be called 'black' rather than 'coloured'. I think they referred to me as 'coloured' at the pre-placement visit. Often staff are scared of saying the wrong word in case they offend, so they don't say anything. People here seem to think it is derogatory to use the term 'black'."

One student recalled an encounter she had with a home-help organiser:

> "She said to me 'Where do you come from?' and 'You won't have knowledge of the way we live'. I said 'Excuse me, I have been in this country for 20 years – I was educated here and I work here'. However, I think it was because I was challenging her decision about a client."

She continued:

> "I personally feel that if you don't challenge attitudes then there isn't going to be any change, but it is important to do it constructively if you can. But if you didn't have the confidence you would probably let it go, but then the [racist] attitudes would prevail."

However, black students who were new to social work practice were much less confident, and felt extremely vulnerable in dealing with racism that they experienced. It was made worse when their practice teachers lacked knowledge and awareness.

One student found it very difficult when a senior social worker made derogatory comments to her regarding Salman Rushdie. She stated that:

> "It has not been dealt with satisfactorily. I don't really know whether to complain about it or not. I have spoken to my family who told me to raise it with my practice teacher, and I have also talked to my tutor. You see, I worry about raising questions about 'race' because you don't know how other people are going to react. But if you know people have an understanding of 'race' and culture then it really helps, as you feel you can speak about things more freely."

An elderly client, who also said she came from the kind of country that 'smells', referred to the same student as 'darkie'. The student replied:

> "When the man made the racist remark, the social worker who was with me didn't say anything. I suppose it is easier to take because he is an elderly man who is suffering from dementia. I feel it is much worse when other social workers make comments."

The same student was also faced with challenging cultural stereotypes around religion and arranged marriages. However, towards the end of her placement she said:

"It would really help to have support around these issues, but social workers don't appear to have had any training which is probably why they just ignore it or 'brush it off'."

Another student discussed his experiences, which, despite his past experience, he felt unable to deal with:

"I hear racist jokes in this agency, but I keep my mouth shut. Although it is unacceptable I was not surprised to hear it. I have also had racial taunts from prisoners, but I can accept that more than I can racism from professionals."

He did, however, express the anxiety he felt when he failed to address racist comments and attitudes:

"I just want to get on with my placement, and I don't want any conflict. I know I should raise issues, but I want to pass my course so I keep quiet. But it creates a conflict for me and I feel 'chewed up inside'. I don't know what the outcome would be in the agency. I should have the right to raise these issues, but I am in a vulnerable position. I think it should have been discussed before I started my placement, and I also think we need more black staff in social work."

Another student expressed similar concerns when she said:

"My practice teacher makes subtle racist and sexist jokes, but he just gets away with it because people say 'Oh, it's just his personality'. I used to try to pick him up on things at first, but I am vulnerable and he began saying things like 'Oh well, I don't know if you are going to pass', which made me even more vulnerable."

There were, however, two cases where black students felt able to discuss issues of racism in a constructive manner, without fear of repercussions. One student gave an account of why this was the case:

"I could talk to my practice teacher. I knew early on that I would be fine, as she telephoned me before I came here, said she knew I was black, and we discussed issues related to the fact that I am black. We discussed the issue of dealing with racism at my pre-placement visit, and I was assured I would be supported."

White students also gave accounts of the difficulties that they experienced when they faced racist incidents while on placement. Again, their ability to deal with discrimination was dependent on personal strengths, professional experience, political awareness and the support of their practice teacher. For many, the academic component of the course, with its emphasis on anti-racist practice, was the first time they were faced with addressing the issue. In common with black students, they were also concerned that challenging racism within agencies not aware and/or sympathetic to the issues could have a negative impact on their experiences and their success.

Although one student was initially confident that she would be able to respond constructively to discriminatory incidents or attitudes, when she said "I would deal with it through management", as her placement progressed she became less confident, when she stated that:

> "It would be a problem to raise the issues here, and I would not know what to do because of the general apathy and the power within the management team."

Several other students, who had also become less secure by the end of their placements, repeated her initial response.

Another student who was concerned about racism demonstrated her lack of security in addressing it:

> "I have heard racist and sexist jokes here and I never manage to say anything back. I could try to contact my tutor, because even if you cannot handle it, it helps to talk about it. A hospital worker I was in contact with made a racist comment, and well, I didn't say anything, which I hope, let him know that I wasn't happy. I hope I got the message across because I did not react. It creates personal dilemmas for me all the time."

One student, who was politically committed, confident and experienced, nevertheless had difficulties due to the hostility of her practice teacher to anti-discriminatory issues. She also found other staff seemingly unable or unwilling to deal with issues. She said:

> "I would not feel confident dealing with racism in this agency, mainly because of where the power lies, and I don't think there would be any interest. Other social workers seem to be aware of how awful things are, but don't feel able to do anything about it. So, you get on

with your work and do the best you can. You see, any discriminatory comments are likely to come from my practice teacher. He has made comments that he thinks equal opportunities policies are a waste of time. He keeps calling me 'young lady', and I feel I am going to have to say something soon. He has the view that clients are all scroungers. Early on in my placement I got a referral and showed it to another social worker who said 'Oh, that address, they are all a load of scroungers'. In relation to another case my practice teacher said 'Well, they will be after something, and you go out to see them with two thoughts in mind – they are getting nothing from us financially and their kids are not coming into care'. So, he had written them off before I had chance to speak to them."

Another committed student said:

"It's hard being in the university and having a group of like-minded people. You see in the university you can be more politically active or idealistic, but then you come into an agency, and there are problems with where the power lies. In the end you have to rely on your own support networks."

Several students who were less experienced and less confident, were shocked at the levels of discrimination that they encountered in agencies, especially as most of it came from social work staff. One student said:

"There are racist and sexist attitudes here – things have been said that have horrified me. It is not that they don't affect me, as they do, but the racist attitudes are not directed at me. I have heard [racist] things said here and have been cringing inside. It has made me think, how would black workers be affected. The things said are usually made by staff about staff. I am not sure if the problem is that workers just get used to it, and begin to accept it. I got this silly idea that all social workers would have socialist attitudes and be Left-wing, and unfortunately it is not the reality. Things have been said by senior social workers which I have found difficult to listen to ... but it could alienate you if you disagree. There is no way I could ever work here."

Later in her placement she discussed how she had attempted to deal with racism, and said:

"I try to deal with it in humour, and if I hear someone say something racist, I say 'Right, that is another one down to discuss at the university'. It is not the best way to deal with it, but I feel I am pointing out that I have noticed what they say. But I feel so vulnerable."

Other students also expressed feelings of vulnerability, for example stating that:

"They are giving up some of their time to train me so I certainly don't feel I can go in and criticise their way of working just to get something 'off my chest'. I would rather keep quiet about things, but if I did ask questions [around discrimination] it would be in a non-confrontational and non-threatening way.... But there are lots of little things that you let go that possibly you shouldn't."

Another student said:

"When things have been said that I feel are racist, I try to get a second opinion from one of my colleagues, to make sure that I am not overreacting. That can determine if I take it seriously."

The accounts of both black and white students regarding dealing with racism and discrimination give cause for concern. They reveal the enormous difficulty that all students have in addressing levels of discrimination, and the negative consequences for their social work training. Their inability to deal with discrimination can lead to feelings of anxiety, guilt and disillusionment, especially among students politically and personally committed to anti-discriminatory practice. The implications are more serious for black students, who often feel isolated regarding the racism that they experience, and their attempts to respond to it effectively. There is also evidence that when they do attempt to put such issues on the agenda, they constantly deliberate, assessing the projected response of other agency staff. Almost all students felt that challenging racism might negatively affect their relationship with other staff, their progress, and ultimately their successful completion of placements. The only real exceptions were the experiences of two confident, relatively experienced black students who were in agencies with supportive and radical practice teachers.

The responses of students reveal several important issues. First, the students articulated a variety of strategies for dealing with racism. Initially, they reflected a degree of confidence in the agencies and their management structures to deal with the manifestation of racism, particularly overt racist abuse. A number of students indicated initially that they would consult with management if they came across any racist incidents. In a sense, this managerial response is not surprising. Students who were on placement for the first time had been assured that anti-racism and anti-oppressive social work practice were high on the CCETSW, university and agency agenda, and initially expected agencies and agency management to pursue and tackle all manifestations of racism. However, while on placement, most students became disillusioned in the ability and willingness of management to tackle racism. In the absence of any active management commitment, students adopted a variety of strategies, from confrontation to 'education', from an obvious and deliberate 'ignoring' of comments to show displeasure, to laughing comments off in a way that drew attention to the inappropriateness of what had been said. Each of these represented an individual response to dealing with racism, in the context of having to pass their placement experience in order to qualify as social workers. The immense pressure this placed on students to 'conform', ignore or downplay racism cannot be underestimated. The institutional culture in many agencies was clearly one that supported a racist agenda, for, although racist jokes and comments were not daily occurrences, they did appear to be common enough not to be abnormal or draw general disapproval.

Although the racism that students were subject to within agencies came mainly from a minority of staff, it nevertheless created an atmosphere and culture where racism was, to some degree, legitimated. However, the main problem that students faced from most staff was a lack of confidence, knowledge and awareness in dealing with racism, which often reflected an agency and management culture uncommitted to and/or unaware of the issues. Yet the experiences of several students emphasised that, with the support of practice teachers, a strong black social work presence, and a more conducive anti-racist work culture, it was possible for students (and other workers) to tackle racism within the workplace and from clients. Dealing with racism, and implementing anti-racist social work need to be integrated into the daily working experience, and there is a need for ongoing training for all staff regarding issues of 'race', racism and discrimination. Again, rather than leaving training to agencies with, at best, variable procedures in dealing with racism and providing anti-racist social work practice, there is a need for greater theoretical clarity of 'race' issues and models of countering racism.

FIVE

Implementing anti-racist learning requirements – the importance of the student/practice teacher relationship

It became increasingly evident as interviews with students progressed that the relationship with the practice teacher was the most important factor in determining a student's general experiences on placement, and also their ability to address issues of 'race' and anti-racist social work practice. As noted earlier, Paper 26.3 of the Rules and Regulations for the Diploma in Social Work charged practice teachers with a significant responsibility in facilitating anti-oppressive social work practice, of theorising anti-racist practice, and of keeping up with theoretical debates and developments in this area.

Practice teachers have a great deal of influence in structuring the placement experiences of students and their learning opportunities, and ultimately they are responsible for assessing whether students pass or fail their placements. As such, they have a great deal of power in determining to what extent issues of anti-racist practice reach the placement agenda. The practice teachers interviewed as part of this research project had little knowledge or awareness about 'race' and the implementation of anti-racist practice, and many of them exhibited varying degrees of anxiousness and defensiveness when the issues were raised. Many students differentiated between what they called 'traditional' (or conservative) and 'radical' practice teachers (see the discussion in Chapter Two). They felt that the more 'radical' social workers and practice teachers were 'open' to anti-racist social work practice and more concerned about other forms of discrimination in social work departments. Conversely, conservative practice teachers tended to be more hostile and defensive, not just about 'race', but about a diverse set of oppressions and systemic disadvantages.

The ability of students to share fears, anxieties, difficulties and areas of vulnerability was of vital importance in determining their ability to discuss anti-racist social work theories and practice while on placement.

Dealing with racism was dependent on their practice teacher's knowledge, awareness and commitment to issues of 'race' and anti-racist practice, but even those practice teachers who lacked such knowledge could still be supportive by demonstrating a willingness to be receptive to, and take seriously, confrontations with racism. When practice teachers demonstrate such attributes, students can feel comfortable about the issues despite negative agency cultures and the sometimes hostile attitudes of other staff.

If students had a positive relationship with their practice teacher, then it was possible for them both to work through 'institutional barriers' as positively as possible. The student's experience became more positive even though the agency's practice and culture remained deeply and institutionally racist. Conversely, students with hostile practice teachers or those who had neither the confidence nor knowledge to deal with aspects of anti-oppressive practice, found the institutional barriers insurmountable.

This section will explore the practice teacher/student relationship from students' perspectives in the following way. First, we will look at students with conservative practice teachers who, in general, had negative placement experiences. Second, students with social democratic practice teachers tended to have positive experiences in relation to general practice, but negative experiences regarding anti-racist social work practice. Last, students with radical practice teachers tended to have positive experiences in all aspects of their placement practice.

The terms 'positive' and 'negative' are used here to refer to the practice teacher's ability and interest in facilitating anti-oppressive practice. Conservative practice teachers were hostile to anti-discriminatory initiatives, were not interested in developing their skills, knowledge and awareness in this area, and tended to respond negatively to students experiencing difficulties, often perceiving them as arising from personal deficiencies. In general, the student placement was negative, and this was reinforced with regard to anti-oppressive practice. The majority of social democratic practice teachers were not overtly hostile to anti-discriminatory issues, but were unable to facilitate anti-racist learning requirements, or to support students adequately around issues of discrimination, due to lack of knowledge and awareness, and/or feelings of vulnerability. In some instances this led to a denial or undermining of the experiences of students, and in these areas the placement was negative. Radical social workers tended to be 'open' to new theories and developments, particularly in relation to anti-discriminatory practice, and were willing to recognise and act on gaps in their own practice, knowledge and awareness. Their students felt more able to share their fears, experiences and areas of weakness while on placement, and were more likely to be given credit for the strengths they brought to social work practice. They also legitimised rather than dismissed any difficulties students were experiencing. These factors made the overall placement experience much more positive.

Student relationships with conservative practice teachers

Earlier, conservative practice teachers were identified as holding a variety of familial, pathologising and controlling perspectives on social work's role in society. These practitioners also tended to view social work as a 'practical', atheoretical activity, rather than a knowledge-based activity. As a consequence, they were generally hostile to the emphases of anti-oppressive social work. Perhaps ironically, given their emphasis on 'practice', students with conservative practice teachers reported the most negative placement experiences. The accounts of black students will be explored first:

> "I don't really feel comfortable with him; he comes over as a chauvinistic type of person, which was confirmed by other female workers. I don't feel that he is aware of issues of 'race' and gender although he says he is. I feel more comfortable knowing that other workers share my views, although they seem to have got used to it.... But issues of 'race' are not addressed, and if I bring them up I get the impression that he is thinking 'Oh no, she is bringing that up again'."

> "My practice teacher takes things very personally, and is over-sensitive about a lot of things. She is not overtly nasty, but she is hostile to criticism and does not see it as something to improve things. I think she saw me as a threat which was awful, as I was there to learn."

> "I have been mainly left to get on with things and my practice teacher doesn't seem sensitive to the needs of students. We rarely talk about anti-discriminatory issues and I don't raise them as they might be held against me."

In the atmosphere of the placement, the students were either expected to practice and ignore 'personal agendas' around the implementation of theory and anti-oppressive practice, or to establish strategies to counter the various inequalities faced by clients.

White students were also negatively affected by the attitudes and approaches of conservative practice teachers. One student spoke at great length of her dissatisfaction with her practice teacher:

> "He was not interested in the pre-placement contract and he tends to think that education is a waste of time. It seems to me that he wants a social work assistant because he is short-staffed. He hasn't given me much time and I feel very unsupported. I consider him to be my biggest problem and I am just going through the motions with him. He hasn't shown any interest when things have got difficult for me, and has avoided me. He is on a different 'wavelength' and he seems to see having a student as a bit of an 'ego trip'. I have given up trying to discuss things with him.... I know that he would not take on board anti-racist issues. When I mentioned it, he said he wasn't interested in 'banner waving'. He is hostile to any issues of inequality and it is reflected in his attitudes and his practices. He is very much of the view that people are 'deserving' or 'undeserving'. I think he chooses to ignore the academic course content and does not have any idea about theories and methods. He has said things like 'Oh, black students get a better deal don't they?'.... It has all been very disappointing as you want your practice teacher to be someone who is aware and wants to change things, rather than being someone who is part of what needs changing."

Another white student stated:

> "It is very difficult having an extremely 'traditional' practice teacher who has been in the job for years and has not moved on. She sees people who come in with new ideas and enthusiasm as a threat, so my placement has gone against everything I have learnt at college in relation to progressive thinking."

Although the institutional and structural nature of racism in society is a key and central determinant shaping black people's lives, this does not mean that individual actions and attitudes are unimportant. Individual prejudices can have direct consequences on others, especially when those individuals are in positions of relative authority. Practice teachers were given a key role in CCETSW's developments but this meant hostile practice teachers could have a detrimental impact on students' experiences and their ability to develop and implement their anti-oppressive practice. These practice teachers' views on social work education and training were therefore a direct impediment to fulfilling CCETSW's goal.

Student relationships with social democratic practice teachers

Social democratic social workers are identified as representing the majority of practitioners. They are committed to democratic notions of equality, justice and gradual reform and improvement of life under modern capitalism. For most students, relationships with social democratic practice teachers were generally positive, except in the area of anti-racist practice. Most practice teachers appeared to lack knowledge and awareness in this area, which left them feeling inadequate and insecure. As a result, students were not able to discuss openly issues associated with 'race' and racism, and their experiences of racism were denied or undermined, and consequently not dealt with appropriately. For example, one female black student had a very positive relationship with her practice teacher, but the racism that she experienced was never addressed satisfactorily or resolved, due to her practice teacher's failure to take any constructive action. The student said:

> "I have talked to my practice teacher about offensive remarks made to me while I have been here and I said I didn't think it was acceptable. She said she would try to get one social worker to apologise, and if anything else happens I should go back to her."

The student was also concerned that, despite her personal experiences of racism, her practice teacher, in a meeting with other practice teachers, denied the need for anti-racist training. She observed:

> "At a recent practice teacher's meeting they were saying that 'race' and racism should be taken on board as issues affecting students, but my practice teacher did not agree. I asked her why and she said that the people who she worked with were not racist. I said, 'What about my experiences?' and she just replied, 'Well, if anyone else says anything bad to you we will do something about it'."

This was an incident where, despite evidence of overt racism, the student's practice teacher still denied the need for anti-racist training, and was instrumental in undermining her experiences of racism. As a result, as the placement progressed, this particular student began colluding with her practice teacher's interpretation of racism in agencies. For example, in relation to a racist remark she encountered from a senior social worker, which she initially challenged her practice teacher about, by the end of her placement her interpretation was:

> "Well, my practice teacher and I have come to the conclusion that he was only joking and it was enough that he himself knew he was wrong."

Also, in relation to a racist incident with an elderly client, she said, "Well, he probably didn't know what he was saying, and there is not much anyone can do anyway". It became clear as her placement progressed that she almost 'gave up' attempting to challenge or discuss the racism that she experienced, as there was little recognition or support from her practice teacher, and she did not want to jeopardise the positive relationship they had in other aspects of practice. There were too many risks involved in raising issues around 'race' and racism, and collusion became a more productive and less threatening strategy.

Other students also described feelings of vulnerability in raising anti-racist issues, despite experiencing positive relationships with their practice teachers in other areas of work. One experienced black student said that she attempted to raise issues around racism in a way that would not appear challenging or threatening to other agency staff, so that her contributions would be regarded as positive and constructive. However, her practice teacher had from the start said that he felt he lacked knowledge and awareness of anti-racist practice. Another student was also warned by his practice teacher that some of the staff in the agency were racist, but he was not adequately supported when he experienced racism.

Another white student was aware that her practice teacher appeared apprehensive about anti-racist practice when she said:

> "My practice teacher is very supportive and although she is not particularly aware of anti-discriminatory issues she is interested in learning, and she has said that she has learnt from my input which is nice. But when I began the placement she said, 'You do a lot on

anti-racist practice at the university don't you?' and she appeared quite threatened by it."

There were other white students who, while experiencing generally positive relationships with their practice teachers, were nevertheless concerned about discussing anti-discriminatory issues. For example, one said:

"We have a very open and honest relationship, but I have felt at times that there are some things that have been tricky to bring up, and that some areas of debate are a bit too confrontational."

Another stated that:

"I get on well with my practice teacher and other staff, but I think they feel I am fresh from college with my new ideas which are idealistic and naïve, ideas which are promoted in the university regarding 'race', gender and class."

A student who was jointly supervised in a mainly positive way by two practice teachers nevertheless said that she preferred one of them because "he is very strong on inequalities and is aware of issues around inequality". Another said, "My practice teacher seems sincere and caring about social work but I am not convinced that she is 'on the ball' with anti-discrimination".

The majority of practice teachers covered in the research fell into the categorisation of 'social democratic' social workers. They took their role seriously, were generally supportive and were prepared to engage with the students' concerns, but issues of 'race' and racism were avoided, ignored, dismissed or, at best, addressed in an ad hoc manner. These practice teachers were not hardened racists – far from it – but lack of resources and the absence of appropriate training left them feeling inadequately prepared to meet the students' needs or to be able to confidently confront racist practice or the dominant culture of institutional racism. In the absence of such resources and training, and in a growing climate of backlash (see Chapter Seven), practice teachers resorted to various avoidance strategies.

Student relationships with radical practice teachers

Radical practitioners were those that were identified as locating their client's problems within the social structure and the range of oppressive practices dominant in society. Consequently, these social workers were more open to a range of anti-oppressive initiatives. The students who experienced the most positive placement experiences were those with radical practice teachers. For example, one black student who had a more conservative practice teacher during her first placement described the difference it made to have a radical practice teacher on her second. She said:

> "My practice teacher is about my age and I can talk to her about most things and she understands. She only qualified three years ago, but I feel supported by her both personally and professionally.... Last year there was no knowledge at all about 'race' and racism from my practice teacher ... she had no idea. When I discussed racism she would say things like 'Nothing is that bad, surely' and 'I don't believe people think things like that'. This year my practice teacher understands the issues, and I have come to the conclusion that social workers who are not sensitive to the issues should not be allowed to have students. My practice teacher is quite interested in black art and culture, and I don't know where she picked it all up, but she knows exactly what I am talking about, whereas last year there was no acceptance of what I was saying. She also recognises the importance of black support groups and encourages me to go. My last practice teacher was very defensive and if I had gone to a black support group she would have thought I was plotting against her."

Another black student also compared his relationship with different practice teachers:

> "Last year my relationship with my practice teacher was good, but there was a lot of racism and he was not always around to support me. This practice teacher has a good approach to 'race' and we discusses issues of equality associated with sexuality, 'race', gender and the rights of clients."

He also described how he was offered opportunities to work with black and gay clients and was assisted in providing sensitive and appropriate services by his practice teacher, who discussed issues freely with him. His practice teacher was also prepared to learn from him, and this increased his confidence in raising issues around racism. Other students also discussed relationships with more radical practice teachers, making comments such as, "My last practice teacher was open-minded but had a lot of conservative ideas, whereas this practice teacher has been brought up in my time". Another black student spoke at length of his positive relationship with his practice teacher:

> "I am very happy with this relationship. She is my type of person with a radical approach to social work that is much different from the more traditional type of social worker. She is concerned with injustices. When I was relatively new to social work, I used to follow the practice of other social workers, but looking back at the kind of professionals they were, I would dread it if I had a more traditional practice teacher. Traditional practice teachers still have a view of clients who should 'get off their backsides', and they don't take into account the injustice and inequality in society. Our lives are not always determined by our own actions, but by the actions of others. That is a plus point for the university, as it does prepare students for social work that recognises this. I don't mean the radical 'loony-Left' type preparation, but radical with a lot of theoretical knowledge. But then there are problems if you get a traditional practice teacher – I've heard of awful clashes. You have almost got to have similar political views because social work is so politically oriented. My practice teacher and I have stimulating discussions and respect each other's views even if we don't agree all the time. She has worked with black staff and clients in the past, and is very knowledgeable. She is learning Urdu at the moment because there is a very high Asian population in this town, and she feels it might help her to communicate better with sections of the community."

This student's experience was positive as a result of compatible professional approaches to social work, a secure learning environment, the structural contextualisation of social work issues and a relationship which was based on open and honest explorations of theory and practice, especially around anti-discriminatory issues.

For all students, two aspects of the placement experience that were important in raising issues regarding anti-discriminatory practice were supervision sessions and the pre-placement meeting. Both were forums that, if used constructively, gave students an opportunity to discuss their experiences of discrimination, explore the implementation of anti-racist practice, and link theory and practice. They are discussed briefly below.

Supervision sessions

Supervision sessions involve students and practice teachers meeting to discuss caseloads and progress. Although the research revealed enormous disparities in students' experiences, actual approaches to supervision can be broadly divided into two categories: a functional approach to supervision and an investigative/theoretical approach. Issues such as time available and regularity of supervision sessions compound both approaches.

Generally, the supervision sessions were negatively affected as a consequence of workloads and time demands placed on practice teachers. Lengthy sessions with students were often a 'luxury' that many practice teachers could not afford, especially when agencies offered little in the way of reduced workloads. Despite this there were some excellent examples of good practice. The best examples of supervision in terms of student feedback were those that were regular weekly events, planned and timed in advance, and where the themes covered were a wide review of theoretical and practical issues and concerns. These sessions became positive learning experiences where the difficulties of applying theory to practice were discussed and debated. Here, the supervision sessions became a bridge between the academic component in the university and practice in the field. The investigative/theoretical approach to supervision was more likely to be practised by radical practice teachers, who tended to be more recently qualified and more open to new ideas and developments. This approach does plan for, explore and assess specific cases in relation to client intervention, but it then takes the discussion and analysis forward by incorporating wider psychological, theoretical and ideological debates. Students' personal feelings, emotions and insecurities are also more likely to be explored in a supportive learning environment. Here supervision is more likely to become a two-way process, with practice teachers willing to learn from and acknowledge the strengths and abilities that students bring to the placement experience. This again is particularly important for black students' experiences on placement, and the willingness of practice teachers to acknowledge the racism that they experience in all aspects of their lives. This approach to supervision is more conducive to enabling students to realise their full potential and also assists students in broadening and expanding their knowledge, understanding and expertise.

In terms of regularity of supervision sessions, it was radical and social democratic practice teachers who tended to give more time and commitment to supervision to ensure that a decent amount of time was set aside for discussion. Although, even when social democratic practice teachers attempted to structure sessions around issues of anti-oppression, there was some indication that they were uncertain about the exact nature of anti-racist social work. It seemed reduced, in some well-meaning cases, to a form of cultural awareness or multiculturalism. However, this was an improvement on the lack of help, support and advice available to many students from their practice teachers.

It was those practice teachers who were more conservative in their approach who tended to ignore the needs of students in terms of regular time slots set aside for supervision. Their students often had to rely on past professional experience and feedback from other staff in order to assess their relative success.

The worst examples occurred when supervision sessions were irregular, badly planned and formalistic. Theoretical issues and problems were not raised and discussed, and practice teachers leading these sessions utilised the time merely to review work undertaken. The sessions then became, at best, a functional device to enable teachers to recognise gaps in the student's experience, or worse, to find out what the students had been doing.

These practice teachers tended to be those who had been qualified the longest, and they tended to favour a functionalist approach to supervision. This approach is characterised by supervision sessions which basically plan strategies of client intervention, and then review the success or failure of that intervention. This approach fails to explore in detail how or why intervention was successful or unsuccessful, and students' feelings regarding their experiences. There is no incorporation of wider social, political and ideological debates and theories regarding the nature of social work intervention and the nature of client group representation. As such, there is no forum for exploring 'race' and racism in society and its reflection in social work departments. The consequence is that there is increasing, subtle pressure on students to conform to existing work norms, not to raise awkward issues and questions, and to get on with the job 'as it is'. Here we see a brief snapshot of the pressures towards the 'incorporation' of students and staff to existing agency procedures, norms and practices.

Finally, it is worth reiterating that for CCETSW's anti-racist initiative, the practice teacher's role and the educative and learning 'bridge' potentially offered by supervision was generally not being fulfilled. For the agencies the evidence revealed a lack of concern and seriousness over student education and training. The de-prioritisation of student supervision revealed an unwillingness to change and confront existing practices, even when these were shown to be oppressive, an inability to engage with theoretical developments in the field, and a failure to give adequate support to both students and practice teachers (who rarely had appropriately reduced caseloads). Given this evidence, moves towards a more practical social work training devoid of any academic input from the social sciences is a great concern.

Placement preparation

The research revealed that discussion over anti-racist learning requirements and dealing with racism was rarely on the pre-placement agenda. Consequently, preparation for placement rarely offered black students the opportunity to discuss dealing with potential racist incidents while on placement. There was little or no discussion about the manifestation of racism in social work and the implications for black students, black staff and black clients, and little recognition of the course content in relation to anti-racist practice. Some responsibility for this situation clearly rests with the university and tutors who should have the experience and appropriate 'distance' from the agency to ensure that the learning outcomes and educative content of placements are prioritised. Yet clearly there was often an awkward relationship between agencies and universities, and university tutors, like practice teachers, also appeared insecure and/or lacked confidence in relation to CCETSW's anti-racist requirements. Again, there was evidence that the precise meaning and form of anti-racist social work was unclear, and what was being promoted in many cases was cultural sensitivity and awareness (if anti-racist issues reached the agenda at pre-placement meetings).

The pressure on university courses to find suitable placements was, and still is, immense, and this could have had an effect on tutors' attitudes to agency practices at pre-placement meetings. However, the failure to incorporate anti-discriminatory debates at this stage of the placement process had serious implications for black students' experiences. The research also revealed that there was enormous pressure on students to take placements even when they felt they were inappropriate to their learning needs, or they were concerned about their practice teacher's attitudes. Some students who experienced late placements had little initial knowledge of the agency they were placed in, or the client groups they would be working with.

There was also evidence from students that practice learning agreements were not always adhered to in terms of achieving learning objectives, and that such agreements were abused in some cases, when students were 'used' as social work assistants. Some students were also much more disadvantaged than others in terms of number of hours worked, and their ability to study and complete written assignments. It was those practice teachers who acknowledged that students were on placement to learn and develop social work skills, and were less hostile to academic and theoretical input, who were more likely to honour study days and be sensitive to hours worked. However, there were practice teachers who were critical of study days and reduced working hours. They tended to view such concessions as privileges rather than positive and necessary learning requirements. As a result, their students often struggled to carry full caseloads while attempting to complete academic work and agency studies, and felt unable to take study days. Their vulnerability and powerlessness often made it very difficult for them to challenge such arrangements, as they felt they would antagonise their practice teachers, and possibly jeopardise their placement success. Because practice learning agreements were often deficient and lacked clarity in relation to learning objectives, support mechanisms and grievance procedures, students relied heavily on their relationship with their practice teacher when difficulties arose.

There were also great differences in students' experiences of 'settling in' to placements. Some agencies and practice teachers appeared much more sensitive than others to familiarising students with agency practices and procedures in a constructive and non-threatening way. However, in other instances, students were literally 'thrown in at the deep end', with little preparation for the work they would be doing. Although experienced and confident students were less susceptible in such incidents, they still found the experience unsettling. The consequences for less experienced students were much more traumatic. Inadequate, unconstructive and insensitive placement preparation had a detrimental effect on all students' experiences.

Both black and white students' accounts of their relationship with their practice teacher expose salient factors that contribute to positive placement experiences. They also reveal factors that contribute to a student's security and confidence in exploring anti-discriminatory theories and practices as part of their learning experiences. As noted earlier, under CCETSW's anti-racist initiative, practice teachers were given a central role in implementing anti-racist social work training, and keeping up with debates and theoretical developments in this area. In effect, practice teachers were being given the role of challenging existing agency practices, and both promoting and developing anti-racist social work in the field, by establishing good practice with students. Yet the evidence presented in this section highlights the problems and limitations that existed with regard to practice teachers fulfilling these aims and being given this role. First, a theme that will be developed later, but is worth noting here, is that practice teachers were being given this significant role at a time when the profession was under political and financial pressures, when the job was becoming more stressful and burdensome, and social work was increasingly a profession 'under siege' (Jones, 1996). Given this context, the extra work and tasks linked to ensuring students could operationalise anti-racist practice could be interpreted as a 'further burden'. This is not to justify a practice teacher's lack of interest, apathy or hostility to this area of work. Indeed, the fact that some practice teachers could and did facilitate anti-racist practice shows that it was possible. Nevertheless, the general context is one important factor that needs to be taken into account. Second, the Diploma of Social Work's recognition of Britain as a structurally racist society was an important development that allowed fuller recognition of the context within which social work, as an activity, takes place. However, this perspective is not one that the majority of the population in Britain would adhere to, nor one that the majority of social workers would advance. Of course, theoretical perspectives need to move beyond common sense understandings and challenge unquestioned norms of social living. But the perspective CCETSW endorsed within the Diploma was imposed on practice teachers drawn from a range of agencies, with differing political views and understandings of their role as social workers, and from different occupational locations within the social work management hierarchy. For practice teachers to be in a position to enable students to fulfil anti-racist requirements required more than simply imposing a 'radical world view'. Instead, the perspective needed to be 'won' through argument, education and the ongoing training of practice teachers.

As we have noted already, social work is not an homogenous profession, but incorporates people with a range of perspectives and outlooks on the world, and a variety of interpretations regarding the function of social work in society, and their role as social workers. Traditional or conservative social workers include people who combine a wide variety of broadly conservative and social democratic concerns regarding the function and justification of both social work as a macro-level enterprise and, at a micro-level, their social work practice. As a consequence, traditional practice teachers are less likely to be receptive to progressive developments, especially in relation to anti-discriminatory practice. They appear to have a more utilitarian approach to social work intervention and expect students to practice in a way that is compatible with agency norms, which is often incompatible with anti-racist practice. Placements are more likely to be perceived as work experiences rather than learning experiences, and students are often denied the time, space and learning environment that they need in order to develop social work skills. Some of the traditional practice teachers were hostile to CCETSW's developments, and dismissive of the need for anti-oppressive practice. Others were overtly racist. But for many it was more that they felt threatened by new methods and theories. In contrast, radical social workers were more receptive to progressive social work developments, including the introduction of anti-discriminatory practices and the implementation of anti-racist theories. They were less defensive about such developments, and felt less threatened by students challenging established practices and values.

SIX

Practice teachers and anti-racist social work practice

The previous two chapters have revealed the extent to which students were dependent on the support of their practice teachers while on placement, particularly in relation to developing and implementing CCETSW's anti-racist requirements. The evidence, however, revealed that only a minority of students felt that their practice teachers were receptive and sympathetic to anti-racist developments. Most others were not confident that practice teachers had the knowledge, awareness or understanding to facilitate anti-oppressive practice, and in some cases felt they were overtly hostile to the issues. As well as interviewing students, the research project involved interviews with each student's practice teacher once during the placement process. The purpose of these interviews was to explore if they were aware of CCETSW's anti-racist programme, if agencies were able to facilitate anti-racist learning opportunities, and if there were institutional barriers to CCETSW's developments.

Their responses revealed that none had experienced any substantial education or training in the field of anti-racist practice, which had serious consequences for students, but also had negative implications for the experiences of practice teachers themselves. For example, most had never explored 'race', racism and anti-racist practice, but were nevertheless expected to undertake anti-discriminatory supervision with little or no constructive preparation or agency support. This led to a situation where many practice teachers felt vulnerable, threatened and confused in relation to both black student supervision and anti-racist practice. Another barrier appeared to be the fear of practice teachers that to display such vulnerabilities could challenge their personal and professional credentials. As a result, it was only those practice teachers who had a personal commitment to anti-discriminatory practice who were confident in facilitating anti-racist supervision. However, due to the lack of institutional and professional commitment to the issues, this group of practice teachers were also susceptible to feelings of insecurity and isolation.

The first part of this chapter explores the accounts of practice teachers who supervised black students. For the majority of practice teachers it was the first time that they had supervised or worked with black students, and very few appeared to have worked with other black social workers or clients. For many, therefore, it was the first time they were confronted directly and indirectly with anti-racist issues.

Supervising black students

There was only one practice teacher supervising a black student who appeared personally hostile to anti-racist social work practice, but his attitude revealed the detrimental impact on the experiences of his student. As well as being negative, his account was also confusing and contradictory, a situation that was not unusual among other practice teachers. He said in relation to issues of 'race' and racism:

> "I don't think racism is important because this agency has been working with black people for a number of years.... It depends where you are coming from. If you have not seen many black people then you tend to be racist, but as you get more involved with them and you know more, the less racist you become if that is your choice."

When questioned about his relationship with his student, he said:

> "Individuals bring themselves to the job and they have their own problems. Now it may well be that because this student has been black all her life she has learnt a range of mechanisms for coping with that, and so it may not be a problem for her. I think she presents herself in a way that is not a problem for anyone else. However, I know a man who has a problem being black and he becomes a problem for other people, but I am not sure if it is his psychological makeup."

Thus, the problem of racism became reduced to the psychological problems of the victims of discrimination with personal adaptation to racism the solution on offer to black social workers and clients.

In relation to the ability of agencies to deal effectively with discrimination, he stated that:

> "Well, agencies certainly have prejudices. They don't set out to be racist or sexist, they just use whatever they can to 'keep you in line', and it is the same if you are male, middle-class, black, white or striped.

I think we are all racist in a sense. People of my age have lived through a whole range of immigration policies and all sorts of media rubbish, and we hear throwaway comments about the Irish, for example, which can be abusive. I think I would claim to be racist, but not deliberately so. I would be concerned to change but I am sick to death of having to apologise for what I am. I suppose I would be prepared to make accommodations rather than being referred to as some kind of social leper."

This account raises a myriad of issues and concerns. There appears to be no awareness, sensitivity or validation given to the insecurities and feelings of the student in relation to the possible manifestation of racism and the implications for her own development. Furthermore, it is an account that individualises, problematises and personalises racism, demonstrating no recognition of the structural and institutional oppression of black groups in society, and how this is informed and reinforced by negative stereotypes. In this sense there is no questioning of white agency norms and social work practices, and no legitimation given to the struggle that black students face while on placement.

There are elements of the above account, which are reflected in those of other practice teachers, especially in relation to students 'fitting in' while on placement, not being a 'problem' to other social workers and not 'rocking the boat' in any way. This results in a situation where black students are unable to speak honestly about their experiences and are, at times, forced to collude with the racism that they experience or observe. There is also an indication, again reflected in the accounts of other practice teachers, that they often internalise and personalise suggestions that they may be unintentionally perpetrating racist practices. This tends to lead to hostility, defensiveness and anxiety when supervising black students and working with black clients which, in turn, leads to a paralysis in terms of developing anti-racist practice.

However, the majority of practice teachers who supervised black students were unable to facilitate anti-racist practice, not because of any personal hostility to the issues, but because of, for example, a lack of security, knowledge and awareness. This reflected the lack of anti-racist educational and training opportunities on social work courses, but was also exacerbated by agency practice and procedures that undermined issues of 'race' and which reflected negative stereotypes of black groups. Again this group of responses indicates a need for an institutional commitment to anti-racist practice in social work agencies in order to signify its legitimacy and ensure its effective implementation.

One practice teacher, whose student spoke of experiencing racism within the agency and outside, said:

> "You come across racism at all levels, but I don't feel that I have had any training, support or preparation for dealing with it. Generally speaking things are down on paper, but there is nothing available that would prepare me for any difficulties arising because of racism. It is very difficult and untested ground, and it is a major problem attempting to raise issues if we as social workers are not getting anything constructive from management. As a result the student suffers. Perhaps the practice teacher owes it to the student to be aware of the issues."

This account begins to demonstrate the immense difficulties and insecurities that practice teachers themselves face when there are no constructive guidelines or agency support in dealing with discrimination. The result is a situation where practice teachers may find racism unacceptable and recognise the gaps in their own practice, but are nevertheless unable to support students on placement. Again the notion of 'contradictory consciousness' is important here. With appropriate support, education and training practice teachers may well be able to facilitate anti-racist social work, but in their absence, and in a hostile agency setting, they are likely to succumb to the dominant agency culture, or ignore the issue, and hence leave the dominant culture unchallenged.

Another practice teacher discussed the manifestation of racism in agencies:

> "There are racist staff in this office. It is not always blatant racism as we are supposed to be a caring profession, although there are individuals who you could call blatant racist bigots. But it isn't taken seriously."

He then spoke of the implications for black students:

> "This office is big and intimidating and if you are a black student there are some people who will be extra hostile to you. Then it becomes even more intimidating. The senior social worker here who has responsibility for student supervision asked me about my present student, when he said, 'How is that 'paki' coming on?' This man is a manager and has been handpicked for promotion.... There is also a bloke here who supervises students and talks about 'our

brothers from the Asian sub-continent' all the time. My [black] student told me that he recently played football against a team of social workers from another division, and every time he got the ball he was called a 'black bastard'.... That is why I think the university should have some overall analysis of where they place students. There are some social workers here who I would never place a black student with, in fact, I wouldn't place any student with them."

When asked about dealing with the racism that he was aware of, he said:

"People are reluctant to take up grievances because it will result in confrontation with management and the best you would ever get is an apology.... I have attempted to deal with the racism that my student experienced from the senior social worker. I said, 'If you talk to him like that again, I will pick up the phone and there will be trouble'. He blustered a bit, but he is a bit of an idiot who thinks it is the 'norm' to think as he does. That is why you wonder if it is worth challenging things, because the views of some people are entrenched and I am not sure what can be done about it. That is why I feel it is very important to start legislating against it [racism]."

This account again demonstrates the vulnerability and insecurity which practice teachers face when they are expected to deal with racism in ad hoc and individualistic ways. Again, with better support and training, this practice teacher may well have been willing to act with others to isolate racism in the workplace. The contradiction, his evaluation of racism and its negative consequences and his 'hopelessness' that little can be done, could be overcome in a different climate which was supportive and demonstrated a collectivist anti-racist approach. However, until there are constructive institutional developments, the ability of practice teachers to confront racism will be limited.

The above practice teachers, although finding it difficult to deal with racism, did nevertheless acknowledge its manifestation in social work agencies, and in this respect it was on the learning agenda. However, there were other practice teachers supervising black students who tended to deny, undermine and misinterpret the racism evident in their organisations. For example, one black student who experienced racism while on placement and discussed it with her practice teacher found that the incidents were often undermined. In relation to a racist comment made by another social worker, her practice teacher said:

> "I didn't expect any comments like that and I was put on the spot a bit. But I don't think he [the social worker] meant any harm. I think it is just the sort of bloke he is – he is very quick-witted and thinks he is being funny.... My student was also in contact with another man who was talking about 'pakis' but she tried to ignore it and as a result he was very nice and asked her how to pronounce her name."

The account reveals no real recognition of the seriousness of such incidents. This particular practice teacher then undermined the racist incidents further by equating them with the discrimination that she faced because she looked young. She said:

> "I have used my own experiences to let my student know that you are not always the person that clients expect on the doorstep. You see, I used to be discriminated against because I looked young and people used to refer to me as 'a bit of a kid'. So, I have had to put up with discrimination which was not obvious."

However, there were instances when practice teachers were complementary about and impressed by the skills that their black students brought to social work agencies, particularly citing their knowledge of 'race' and social work. For example, one practice teacher stated that:

> "She [the student] has enhanced the team and I have become more open to recognising my lack of awareness around issues of 'race'. She has been able to advise me on some of the cultural aspects of 'race', and my lack of understanding has left me feeling quite inadequate at times. She has definitely raised the awareness of the team."

While not wishing to denigrate this response, it does again seem to indicate that there is confusion between anti-racism and wider 'cultural awareness', something which in itself may be 'worthy', but does not equate with 'anti-racism', defined as the conscious attempt to counter all manifestations of discrimination and inequality based on supposed 'racial' characteristics. The same practice teacher also mentioned the fact that his student was quite 'westernised' and progressive, which made him feel easier about supervising her. While revealing some of his own stereotypes, this also indicates that experienced black students and students who adopt agency work norms are, in many instances, perceived more favourably, and seen as less threatening in social work agencies.

Another practice teacher said:

> "I had an Asian female student last year but she was confused and could not grasp the agency's way of thinking and the way problems were approached. But it hasn't been a problem for this student to grasp the ethos of the agency. He has done a lot of work for social services and I have been very impressed with his knowledge which has been useful to us as an organisation."

However, despite these complementary accounts, both students in question, when interviewed, suggested that they thought there was a fine line between being perceived as constructive and being seen as having a 'chip on your shoulder' within the agency. This was a dilemma that they did not feel able to discuss with their practice teachers.

The lack of confidence and experience social workers have around issues of 'race' and racism means that often black students feel they are being used as 'experts' in relation to 'race' and social work practice. For example, another practice teacher relied heavily on her student for information regarding resources for black clients. She said:

> "We are in a multiracial area and what we have noticed with all these debates coming up in the university is that we have more black people walking around outside. We don't know whether it is because they are moving into the area, or that we have not noticed them before. But we feel more alert now and students have helped us."

Here again there seems to be some confusion over the nature and form of anti-racist social work. Here, 'anti-racism' has apparently become a form of superficial 'consciousness raising' about the existence of a local black community. The account also exposes the dearth of knowledge and awareness surrounding anti-racist practice in many agencies, where issues of 'race' and racism only reach the learning agenda if students put them there. This has worrying implications for prospective black clients who are unlikely to receive sensitive provision when white social workers are ignorant of their circumstances and their needs. It also puts added pressure on black students while they are on placement, or the few black workers in agencies, leading to frustration and insecurity.

There were also a number of instances when practice teachers appeared satisfied that racism would be dealt with constructively in agencies, although their black students were not convinced that this was the case. Again, this was often because there was confusion and ignorance as to what actually constitutes racism, which can be masked when popular racist stereotypes are deployed in social work agencies. There is evidence that until black students and staff are listened to seriously in relation to the racism that affects their personal and professional lives, and appropriate institutional action is taken, their experiences will continue to be ignored or undermined.

Finally, there were also a minority of practice teachers who were able to facilitate anti-racist social work practice mainly because of their personal commitment to anti-discriminatory issues. These practice teachers displayed a sensitivity to issue of 'race' and racism, and also discussed structural discrimination in relation to the black community. One practice teacher had worked extensively with the black community in London and she found black student supervision positive and stimulating:

> "I do not find it a problem supervising black students. I really enjoy it – the different ideas. This area is quite multiracial but different from where I worked in London. Here, there is a large Bengali/Pakistani population and we cover that area, and they suffer from extremely bad social conditions and are a very poor community who do not get a good service from this agency."

> "It was quite different where I worked before, as there was a high Afro-Caribbean population and higher black representation. Racism was much more obvious and oppressive and much easier to get your teeth into. Here, the black population are a disenfranchised community, whereas in London black groups are working with the black population and are getting together and becoming quite assertive. But it is not happening here."

Clearly, locality, the range of political and community resources available to the black community, and the community's own traditions, can have an impact on social work provision. But it is also worth noting that despite this practice teacher's claims, there was a substantial network of 'informal' or 'autonomous' welfare groups within the black community described above. Within the Asian community, cultural and political organisations existed, but there was little contact between these welfare, cultural and political community groups, and the official welfare state and social work agencies. One of the most positive, anti-racist practice teachers, therefore, was perhaps still affected by the agency culture and institutional racism, and did not have knowledge of the local community. This is a point that emphasises the problems individual radical social workers have in a hostile climate.

This particular practice teacher demonstrated an awareness of the difficulties which black students were susceptible to in social work agencies when she said that:

> "When I did my training, students were coming from access courses where they had been well supported, and placed in agencies where they were likely to be criticised, judged, discriminated against and not supported."

She also demonstrated a critical awareness not shared by many practice teachers when discussing the difficulties in dealing with racism in agencies:

> "There should be disciplinary procedures, but I have not seen them, and to be honest I do not know how things would be dealt with here. Workers in this department are not overtly racist and they are quite willing to explore issues. However, I would still feel much less secure raising things here than where I worked before, and if I were a black social worker I would feel less comfortable. However, it could be worse as I am comparing the situation with inner London authorities that are much different."

> "I think ... that black people know how to deal with racism to a point. I don't mean that they shouldn't be protected, but actually that it is something they have experienced for most of their lives. As a result, they usually know their own personal limits of what they can tolerate. So, I guess it becomes a problem after that point, and when it becomes offensive to them or interferes with the work they are doing."

> "If racism were coming from a client then there would come a point where someone in a senior position would have to confront the client, but that can be difficult because you cannot withdraw services. Dealing with racism from colleagues also creates problems, and you have to try to be constructive and positive rather than critical. But I don't think that we should put up with anything aggressive,

although most of the time staff are not going round being deliberately racist. It tends to be just ignorance, defensiveness, or not thinking things through, and those are things that can be tackled in reasonably creative ways."

In contrast to the accounts of many other practice teachers, this was more confident, comprehensive, coherent and encouraging. It was also characterised by a degree of sensitivity to the needs of black students. This level of knowledge and awareness contributed to the positive experience of her student while he was on placement, and enabled him to explore anti-racist practice in a supportive environment. There was also awareness that cultural knowledge was valuable but had its limitations:

"There is not enough knowledge and awareness about other cultures which is disappointing, but it needs to go 'cap-in-hand' with anti-racist approaches in order to be useful. I would not want to see training based solely on cultural issues, which is why it is nice for me to have a black student. I mean it is my first contact in any substantial way with people from Pakistan and Bangladesh and cultural and political issues are very much different from those of people I have worked with from India."

A similar level of awareness was also evident in comments made by another practice teacher, who said:

"There were a lot of problems on the course I did when black students could not get placements, and if they did they were more likely to fail, especially in particular agencies. In terms of the ratios, you just knew there was no way it could be right, and the course eventually formally and informally stopped using certain agencies, which was good."

Both these practice teachers also ensured issues of anti-discriminatory practice were discussed at the pre-placement meeting, and were incorporated into the learning agreement. For example, one of them said:

"We discussed at the pre-placement meeting what we would do if the student came up against racist attitudes. In this office, we would approach the person who was responsible for the racism and see them as having the problem rather than the person experiencing it. We would make it clear that it was not acceptable."

Nevertheless, she was aware from experience that dealing with such issues was often difficult, and recounted a specific incident she had been involved in:

"A while ago I was transferring one of my cases to a black social worker here, and when she left the room for something, the clients said that they were members of the National Front and didn't want a 'coloured' social worker. It was really hard to tell the black social worker what they had said, and then I had the dilemma of how to deal with it. I discussed it with her [the black social worker], and the team leader ended up speaking to the clients and saying, 'Look, this is your attitude and so we are going to allocate you a white social worker, but this is because the black social worker does not want to be and should not have to be exposed to your set of attitudes, and if we didn't legally have to offer you a service, then we would withdraw our support'."

This clearly demonstrates a major dilemma facing a consciously anti-racist practice. If anti-racist practice recognises the structural nature of racism and encapsulates a commitment to transforming social praxis, as Mullard (1991) suggests, to what extent can this be compatible with working with nazi clients whose personal commitments include reinforcing divisions based on 'race', denying 'free speech', promoting the forced repatriation of black people, and supporting violent attacks on members of the black community?

The above account demonstrates the importance of team and management attitudes towards issues of 'race', and how a positive agency culture enables practice teachers to implement anti-racist practice in a supportive environment. Nevertheless, despite a positive agency culture this practice teacher also expressed levels of anxiety in dealing with racism at times. She said:

"There are times in this office when people say things unconsciously, for example stereotypes of the Irish, and people challenge them. But it is very difficult when people are upset about what they have said. That is why it should not be left to individual social workers to challenge things. But, I do believe that with the right input, people can change … the issues are seen as important here, but a number of workers are only just beginning to address them. It can definitely affect practice, as we tend to get involved with black and Asian clients when things have reached crisis point. We are not doing enough to encourage them to come in earlier to discuss problems. The fact that we still have too few black and Asian social workers doesn't help either. I think we should be finding out what we could be doing to encourage black clients to come in and seek help. There are so many isolated Asian women in this area, and the budget has just been cut for the Asian women's refuge. I think we should be doing more outreach work, or researching the problem."

Again, if anti-racist practice includes a commitment to 'transforming' the social world, recognising that social services provision for the black community is lacking, and that black people face discrimination as a consequence of their structural location in a racist society, then it should involve a political commitment from social workers and agencies to 'reject' cuts of this nature, cuts which affect some of the most oppressed groups within society. Traditional social work adapts to the limits and barriers placed on agencies by the various workings and determinants of modern societies, structured as they are by a range of oppressions, but an anti-oppressive social work is surely one that stands with the oppressed to reject attacks on their services – otherwise they collude with the system of structured inequality and disadvantage that creates and maintains such oppression.

Both these 'radical' practice teachers were committed to anti-discriminatory practice, but they were also the most critical about its implementation in social work departments, and about its failure to address sensitively the needs of black students and clients, emphasising the difficulties of implementing anti-racist social work practice in institutionally racist organisations. Conversely, it was practice teachers who were not addressing the issues, who demonstrated satisfaction or complacency regarding anti-discriminatory practice.

Although one other student had a positive relationship with his practice teacher, and was able to discuss issues of 'race' and anti-racist practice in an open and secure learning environment, his experiences were lacking because of his practice teacher's focus on cultural issues, and failure to address the nature of institutional racism. This particular practice teacher observed:

"I have had two Asian students, but with my first one I certainly did not learn as much about cross-cultural issues. I suppose with my first student I was not sure how I would take the cultural aspects on, but I did recognise a clear distinction between the collectivist nature of Asian culture, and the individualist nature of European cultures. It has been a very positive learning experience, but I don't understand all the nuances, and I might have to go through it all again if I take an Afro-Caribbean student."

While there was a willingness to discuss issues of 'race' and culture, and the practice teacher was willing to recognise gaps in his experience, these comments again emphasise a confusion over the nature of anti-racist practice, as compared to a well-meaning multiculturalism.

Supervising white students

Of course issues of 'race' and racism were not intended to be left to black students. Anti-racist practice was to be developed by all students, black and white. Once again, however, white students' experiences were affected by their practice teacher's attitude.

Two practice teachers demonstrated varying degrees of personal hostility to issues of 'race' and racism. For example, one practice teacher, when asked about his confidence in supervising black students, said (very sarcastically):

> "You are not suggesting that black students are deficient in intelligence are you? I really do not understand the question, because if someone is trained for social work in this country, then they should be familiar with the way of life of the majority, even if they themselves have a different way of life."

> "There is a lot of silly 'clap-trap' talked about racism. I know there is racism and that it goes on and I know there is racial prejudice. I am not very fond of Scotsmen so that's racist isn't it? It's like if you are a Lancastrian and are working in Yorkshire, then you get 'a bit of stick' because you are from a different tribe. So, I think if someone is of a *completely different tribe* then they will get some stick, and as long as it is not really nasty then they have got to ride it [author's emphasis]. I have a friend who is West Indian and he has problems from time to time getting admitted to places."

When asked about black client and staff representation he said:

> "Well, we have some little old ladies in the villages here, and if a black face knocked on their door, they would probably be highly suspicious and would be reluctant to let them in. As for clients we have one Caribbean chap who lives here with his family, and we have a Chinese lady, and the Chinese 'chippy' family whose children we have in care. That is all.... It would be damn well impossible to implement anti-racist practice here – I think you would have to send students to Bradford."

It is impossible to describe this account as anything but racist. His attitudes had serious consequences for his white student, especially as she was committed to anti-racist practice. However, his views acted as an impenetrable barrier to her development in this area, and despite her extensive social work experience and her strength of character, she experienced anxiety, stress and insecurity while on placement.

Another practice teacher was hostile to anti-discriminatory developments. She identified the type of black social worker who she thought would be 'successful' in the job:

> "I think it depends on how 'westernised' they are and if they have been brought up in this country. I think they have to know how the indigenous population function, and if they have not lived here long, then they are going to have different needs."

> "We have a Section 11 worker who has been with us for five years and I think we take ethnic minorities in our stride because of what she has taught us. We do have a language problem and do feel that some of our indigenous workers should now be taking some of the ethnic minority clients, but they do not have the language. They can only take the cases with good English, the 'westernised' girls."

Both practice teachers incorporated assimilationist assumptions in their accounts, and spoke about black communities as though they were immigrant populations who had not yet successfully integrated into British society. There was no recognition that the majority of black people have been born in this country and are quite familiar with the 'norms of society'. Both practice teachers also inferred that black people were somehow 'the problem', failing to acknowledge the racism inherent in society that is reflected in social work agencies. As such, there was no awareness of the institutional nature of racism (revealed in their personal accounts), nor was there any recognition of, or concern to, develop anti-racist practice.

Other responses from practice teachers, although not overtly hostile to anti-racist practice, lacked any concrete knowledge or critical awareness about 'race' and racism, and again tended to focus on cultural issues. For example, comments were made such as:

> "I would find it difficult to supervise black students because of cultural differences. I would be wary and would be asking myself what was 'normal' in different cultures. But at the moment I have not had enough time to learn about other cultures, so if I had a student who was culturally oriented, I would have problems.... I find students are quite neurotic about the issues at the moment, saying we have got to have black cases and disabled cases because the university says so. This is difficult because we don't have black clients, not because they are excluded, but because they don't seek out services."

There was only one practice teacher supervising a white student who had any real knowledge and awareness of the implementation of anti-discriminatory practice. Again, this appeared to arise from a personal commitment to the issues. She said:

> "This agency is based in a multicultural area and we have got a number of racist neighbours who are trying to engage our support to stop Asians having a mosque, and we have discussed it quite a lot in staff meetings. We don't agree with them, but we are concerned that we are not too militant in dealing with it, as we don't want to alienate them. However, at the same time, we don't want to collude with them in any way."

> "I am sure there must be racism in agencies at a conscious and unconscious level, but I am not always aware of how it is manifesting itself. I would not assume that because we are an agency that deals with prejudice against the disabled, that there are no racist attitudes here. This is something we have started to discuss since we have had a black worker, as we are a very white organisation. I am concerned that we do not load our black worker with issues as there is a tendency to see her as some type of 'expert' which isn't fair."

This analysis was much more critical and sensitive to the issues than the accounts of other practice teachers supervising white students. The practice teacher was aware of the manifestation of institutional racism, and the nature of racism in the local community. These debates and developments ensured that anti-racist practice was on the agency agenda, and was being explored in a progressive and insightful manner, which enhanced the experience of the student placed in this department.

Anti-racist policies within agencies

The accounts of practice teachers revealed that anti-discriminatory policies were not used in any constructive manner to inform the practice of, or support, students while on placement. Below are some of the responses of practice teachers to questions around their awareness of, or the implementation of, such policies:

> "I have not seen anything written down. I know there are guidelines regarding recruitment."

> "Policies around interviewing are well known but there is little knowledge of policies that would inform day-to-day practice. There may be certain people who know about grievance procedures, but by and large they are not known. This makes it difficult to take up grievances."

> "Policies are not really put into practice as they should be. There is very little direction from management."

> "To be honest, I don't think policies are used. Unless you make someone responsible for developing and monitoring them, and you train social workers to use them, then they will be left on the shelf."

Thus, if there were policies, they remained, at best, a blueprint that had not been integrated into practice. Indeed, such blueprints can also feel like (yet another) managerial imposition, not backed up with education, training or appropriate resources.

There was only one practice teacher who located the formulation and implementation of policies in a structural context, and in her response she explored political factors which affect the development and implementation of policies and social work provision. She also assessed their relative impact on mainly deprived social work clients, and assessed the implications of new-Right policies on the morale of social workers.

"I think it depends on how policies are developed and if people feel they own them. I don't think it is helpful if they are imposed from above, but if people play a part in creating them, they are a positive development. I would think that the process is as important as the end product in changing attitudes and raising people's consciousness. I don't think it would be a problem in this agency as there are a lot of willing people who are struggling with a black community that gets a really raw deal."

"It would be nice if the local authority took the lead in developing policies ... and if we could instigate things in this department. But, it is hard to imagine where the energy would come from, as there are so many other pieces of legislation that we have to respond to. We have also been 'rate-capped' here so within the next two weeks we have to close children's homes and homes for the elderly."

"We are in trouble politically so there is not a chance of new projects, as most developments are being frozen. It is very hard at the moment as we only provide very basic services and the community is a very poor one that needs increasing provision."

This account offers a critique of policies which are imposed 'from above', and their vulnerability in the context of political developments hostile to local state provision, particularly that associated with providing services to the most disadvantaged groups in society. During this period social workers and social work departments were experiencing a sustained attack on their ability to provide services, their role in society, and their professional status. So, despite a staff group potentially sympathetic to anti-racist practice, political pressures prohibited its development. The status of anti-racist initiatives was also damaged in the context of government calls for a return to 'traditional' social work skills and an attack on 'theoretically driven agendas'.

Several practice teachers discussed what they perceived as the best way forward in terms of facilitating their anti-racist learning requirements. For example, a practice teacher who was concerned yet insecure and anxious regarding anti-racist initiatives said:

"I would like training courses where it is stated right from the start that it is alright to ask 'stupid' questions about 'race' and culture. We need to be able to explore the issues in a way that is not aggressive because that can do much more harm. We also need to work towards employing more black workers."

Others stated that although they had attended different training courses, they then had to return to social work agencies that were dismissive of, or hostile to, anti-racist practice. So, there was a conflict between anti-discriminatory education and training and institutional racism within agencies, which affected their ability to develop their practice.

More traditional practice teachers, who had been in the social work profession for many years, were, however, hostile to and denied the need for training and development associated with anti-discriminatory practice. The most unconstructive response came from a practice teacher who demonstrated racist attitudes throughout his interview. He said:

> "I think training would be a waste of time for social workers who should know and understand about discrimination and equality. That is what it is all about, caring for people, looking after them and understanding them. If you need training then what the hell are you doing in social work. Coloured people have a difficult time but we should know about it. Maybe I am a bit more aware than others because I live in a town that resembles Karachi [laughing], and our ethnic minorities are almost a majority, so I live alongside coloured folk. I find some of them quite objectionable, but I find others delightful and pleasant."

Another practice teacher suggested:

> "I don't think that there is anything specific I need around anti-racist training. Racism has not touched my life for a long time in a way that has made me angry or made me feel that I have to think about things. You see, most of the problems we face in social work environments are personal issues and they have nothing to do with 'race'."

For CCETSW, practice teachers were given a key role in establishing anti-racist practice. They were the bridge between the university, CCETSW's anti-racist initiatives and the practice in the profession. Yet this chapter has revealed the wide variation in practice teachers' knowledge and awareness about 'race', racism and anti-racist practice. Their responses revealed two crucial factors. First, the institutional setting and policies and procedures are of vital importance in determining the ability of practice teachers to fully implement anti-racist practice. Overwhelmingly, the agencies involved in the research were apathetic, reluctant about, or hostile to anti-racist initiatives, and there was little time given for practice teachers to undertake training and education in this area. There were few developments to improve contact with local black populations, to open up dialogue with local black groups about their needs or perceptions of social work agencies, or to develop services that would match their needs. When formal anti-discriminatory or equal opportunities policies had been adopted, there was little attempt to operationalise them or even publicise them.

Practice teachers charged with ensuring students could undertake anti-racist social work practice, rarely knew what the agency's formal position was, and even committed practice teachers seemed unsure. In no sense did any social workers feel they 'owned' the anti-discriminatory policy agenda; rather it was something 'external' to them that was formally imposed on their activities. The institutional climate was overwhelmingly one that was reluctant to change or consider new ideas and developments. The working culture and ethos was one that portrayed social work as an atheoretical, decontextualised activity concerned with 'practical' tasks and roles that are best described as 'technicist' in orientation. The major impediment to developing anti-racist social work was clearly the practical, technicist and institutionally racist conduct and ethos of agencies. Thus, very few agencies took anti-discriminatory practice seriously, and in most cases it was negligent or absent in terms of practice and professional development.

Second, the attitudes, values and practices of practice teachers clearly impacts on students' experiences of anti-discriminatory supervision. The practice teachers could broadly be divided into three categories that match the 'ideal' types developed in Chapter Two: conservative, social democratic and radical. A small number of conservative practice teachers were clearly racist. Not only did they operate in ways that reflected institutional racism, but also their personal values were racist. This affected their attitudes to black clients, black staff and students, and white staff and students committed to anti-racism. Some of these individuals were in senior management positions in agencies located in areas with significant black populations, which is clearly an issue of concern.

A second minority were the small group of radical social workers who demonstrated a commitment to anti-racist practice. They were aware of the structural nature of racism, the dominant racist culture within Britain, and the manifestation of institutional racism within social work agencies in terms of the position of black staff and the under-representation of, and inadequate provision for, black clients. As a consequence, they were better placed to support black students on placement. The more committed practice teachers had greater theoretical knowledge and awareness regarding 'race' and racism, which they were attempting to translate into social work practice, although lack of support and educational development meant that even this group was unsure about what an anti-racist social work practice would involve. Nevertheless, they were willing to be actively involved in creating and establishing such practice. As a result, they also tended to be much more optimistic about change and more positive about supervising black students.

The main group consisted of practice teachers who were committed to a variety of social democratic values. They were concerned about issues of social injustice and inequality and were aware of the social causes of many problems. They were conscious of racism in society, often aware of racism within social work, but had little experience, education and training in tackling racism and implementing anti-racist social work practice. In terms of CCETSW's original aims, this group of professionals is vital. It is unlikely, at least in the short term, that the 'openly' racist conservative practice teachers can be convinced of anti-racist orientations and the structural nature of racism. Radical social workers are convinced of the need, at least, to be open to the idea of anti-racist practice, and in this sense they are an important mechanism, or 'vanguard' for raising anti-racism within the profession. The majority, reflecting a variety of broadly social democratic principles, are those who need to be targeted and 'won over'. They reflect, in both their theorisation and practice, a contradictory consciousness in the area of 'race'. They are not, for the most part, openly or overtly racist, and are aware of racism and will often work with black clients to meet their needs in the best possible way. However, their practice and orientation may also act and operate in ways that follow the procedures and norms of their agencies, which, in turn, reflect a range of institutionally racist assumptions. In a contradictory way they may justify their own practice in terms of 'treating all clients the same', referring to a 'race-blind' approach, or by stating that, 'in the present climate the department finds it difficult to meet the needs of all client groups'. Nevertheless, when asked about issues of racism, they acknowledge the particular inequalities and oppression facing the black population. In agency cultures that acknowledged such disadvantage and promoted elements of anti-racism, the context was such that many of the social workers in those institutions felt confident, knowledgeable and willing to deal with racism and issues of 'race'.

This suggests that the development of anti-racist social work needs to challenge the policies, practices and procedures of mainstream social work, and the institutional racism of agencies. Such a challenge must attempt to convince the majority of social workers committed to the values and ideas of a broadly social democratic social work of the structural nature of inequalities such as racism, and that with appropriate ongoing education and training programmes, and an active input from black organisations, black social work support groups and radical social workers, anti-racist social work can start to be developed. Yet, any such recognition must conclude that, while we can strive for anti-racist social work practice, the structural and institutional nature of racism means that any anti-racist social work can never be completely successful (to the extent that it eradicates racism). It will only ever be partial and will need to develop and be 'ongoing' until wider transformations abolish all manifestations of racism in society.

The paucity of anti-racist education and training, and the lack of any coherent institutional commitment, resulted in most practice teachers feeling vulnerable and fearful regarding anti-racist supervision. Practice teachers spoke of their dissatisfaction with agency and management support and the lack of constructive placement preparation, which all led to feelings of inadequacy and isolation. However, even those practice teachers wishing to discuss anti-racist issues in an honest and open manner were unable to do so because of a lack of institutional support and the absence of adequate and effective communication mechanisms. As a result, these issues were often dealt with in ad hoc, individualistic and unconstructive ways.

Finally, those feelings of 'insecurity', 'vulnerability' and 'fearfulness' must be placed in context. In the absence of any commitment to anti-racist social work practice from agencies, and the lack of relevant and ongoing anti-racist education and training for social workers, anti-racism can feel like another imposition, and another critique of social work practice. In a profession at the sharp end of state responses to poverty, inequality and discrimination, faced with mounting social problems, and in an atmosphere of cuts and financial restraints, social work is an increasingly difficult and stressful activity. Making matters worse, social work has become a profession 'under siege' and under political attack from local and national government and the media. In this atmosphere, the political nature of anti-racist social work practice could clearly increase anxiety and feelings of isolation. Anti-racist developments could feel like another imposition from above that leaves social workers in the field exposed to charges of 'political correctness'. Without the appropriate agency commitment, education and support, the difficulties of implementing anti-racist practice can feel 'insurmountable' and 'unrealistic' impositions from CCETSW and the academy, with little connection to the problems facing social workers in the field. It was precisely such concerns that fed into the backlash against Paper 30 in the early 1990s, the subject matter of Chapter Seven.

SEVEN

Backlash against CCETSW's anti-racist initiative

As the last three chapters have emphasised, CCETSW's initiative came up against significant barriers within the social work profession: anti-discriminatory policy was not fully implemented or supported in any real sense; dominant agency practices and norms operated in a range of institutionally racist ways; there was a lack of adequate service provision for the black community and under-representation of black staff; practice teachers were generally unwilling or unable to implement anti-racist practice; there was a professional culture within which students raising anti-racist concerns – and black students in particular – were dismissed or even racially abused. In the early years of its operation, CCETSW's policy faced significant internal hurdles. But the anti-racist initiative also came under increasing scrutiny and met hostility from a range of groups outside of the academy and CCETSW's core policy group. Opposition came from the media, government (both national and local) and from inside the profession itself. The anti-racist initiative was increasingly dismissed as a Left-wing, politically correct dogma with no place in social work education, training and practice. By 1992/93 there was an all out backlash against CCETSW and Paper 30. This chapter deals with these events.

As social work education and training attempted to address the issue of structural and institutional oppression in society, it found itself at the forefront of a political debate about the nature of Britain, racism, social welfare and 'political correctness' (PC). In 1992, Virginia Bottomley, the then Health Minister, took CCETSW to task for too great an emphasis on anti-discrimination in qualifying training, and this set the tone for a series of attacks on CCETSW. Things came to a head in August 1993 when several articles attacking CCETSW appeared in the national press. As Jones (1993) states:

> Over a period of four days, Melanie Phillips in *The Observer*, Robert Pinker in the *Daily Mail* and Brian Appleyard in *The Independent* all had major articles virtually a page in length to lambast social work

courses and to portray CCETSW and Paper 30 as the cause of doctrinaire and abusive anti-racist perspectives. (Jones, 1993, p 10)

These articles led to intervention by both politicians and social work practitioners. There were mixed responses in the letters page of *The Observer* (8 August 1993) to the debate. One contributor stated that:

As a social worker for 16 years I wish I could indignantly deny the allegations about political correctness in social work training made by Melanie Phillips. However, they struck me as all too true, not just at the training level but as management policy in the practice of social work. I am torn between shame on behalf of my profession and relief that its present slavish adherence to rigid dogmas at the expense of intellectual open mindedness has been exposed.

Another critical letter (*The Observer*, 8 August 1993) came from the Director, Plymouth Guild of Community Service who argued that:

Melanie Phillips is to be congratulated for drawing attention to the take-over of the social work training council by a group of fanatics and zealots, obsessed only with race and gender issues and politically correct expressions. Both the training council and institutions running social work courses seem to have lost sight of what social work is all about.

There were also two letters from those who supported CCETSW's anti-racist developments, and a letter from Tony Hall, the Director of CCETSW, which stressed that the developments were not concerned with PC but were seeking to ensure that qualifying social workers are able to work effectively in a multiracial and multicultural society. The same debates were also taking place on the letters page of *Community Care* and *Social Work Today* and demonstrated the highly charged and controversial nature of the subject of anti-racist social work. For example, a principal social worker from Harlow stated in *Social Work Today* (2 April 1992) that he believed "CCETSW is led by the ultra-left pushing their multicultural obsessions". Pinker (1999) added to this when he spoke of the publication of training manuals associated with oppressive practice being:

... replete with the lore and language of political correctness ... they categorically rejected the traditional academic beliefs that you have to win people over by rational persuasion, not emotional arguments, and that 'you must not interfere with other people's freedom of speech/action (even if it is racist/sexist)'. (Pinker, 1999, pp 17-18)

As a result of these criticisms, there were moves to undermine the relevance and importance of CCETSW's anti-racist recommendations. Jeffrey Greenwood, in taking over as Chair of CCETSW in Autumn 1993, defined himself as a supporter of equal opportunities, while publicly committing himself to "rooting out politically correct nonsense" (quoted in *The Independent*, 28 August and 19 November). He then ordered a review of CCETSW's anti-discriminatory policies and Paper 30, and a 'new' Paper 30 was published with the formal commitment to anti-racism dropped.

The debate over political correctness

Part of the debate over Paper 30 was constructed around its supposed PC. This is a perjorative term used to dismiss a range of policies aimed at regulating and regularising relationships between workers in a range of institutions, and between workers and various client groups. Central to these developments were attempts to control the use of various words and terms. In part, this was to eradicate 'hate language' – racist, sexist and homophobic terms of abuse, for example. But it quickly moved beyond this to problematise a range of words, within which PC identified the hidden hand of oppression. There is no doubt that this did lead to some rather silly successes. 'Political correctness' could be described as:

> A trend, a cultural phenomenon, a series of attitudes and practices which are an effect or residue of certain aspects of the movement for black, female and gay liberation ... it is what remains of the gains of the movements of the 1960s and early 1970s. (Molyneux, 1993, pp 43-8)

The social roots of PC lie in those sections of the Left and of black, women's and gay movements which attained positions of relative comfort and/or authority in society (in local government, the equal opportunities community and various equal opportunity jobs, for example), and who attempted to use their positions of authority to impose, for example, limited forms of anti-racist practice 'from above'. Thus, despite the way in which political correctness has been depicted by the Right as the fanatical activity of far–Left subversives, it is an activity based on 'gradualist' or reformist politics. Its aim (primarily) is to proscribe certain forms of speech or language, using 'guilt' to challenge morally linguistic forms, while leaving material inequalities unchallenged.

Political correctness in Britain has been concentrated in areas such as social work, local government and primary education, areas within which Left ideas, especially anti–racist ideas, have a significant presence. These areas of state activity have a strong representation of educated Leftists who hold managerial or semi–managerial posts, and the temptation has been to impose anti–racism from above by means of administrative regulations. This led to some of the more detrimental features of PC, which became more acute in the context of attacks on state welfare organisations and declining resources. In many ways, the controversy around what the media called 'loony Left' councils in the 1980s, was later reflected in what was called the PC controversy.

Notions of PC have been particularly associated with the social work profession, especially in relation to mixed–race adoption. A number of social services have taken a position of total opposition to all 'mixed–race' adoptions. Their well–meaning justification has been that black people experience racism in society, and only black parents can give black children the support they need to deal with this. But, behind this, lie a number of typical 'politically correct' ideas, that all whites are racist and that 'white culture' and 'black culture' are completely distinct and separate entities, each of which is, at least, debatable. As a result, black children languish in children's homes, and the focus on 'skin colour' concedes Right–wing racist arguments that 'race' is a fundamental division in society, and that it is impossible for black and white to live together.

Political correctness faced its greatest notoriety and ridicule around its attempts to promote speech codes and language reform. During the 1980s there were moves to tackle racism and bigotry by making it a disciplinary offence to use offensive and abusive language regarding 'race', gender and sexual orientation. Such attempts were attacked by the Right and the media as a violation of free speech.

Language, of course, is always changing and developing. But these reforms involved discovering pejorative or oppressive meanings in words, and attempting to replace them with new, often artificially created expressions. In part, this is based on a vast overestimation of the role of language in bringing about social change, and displays attempts to substitute language for real reform. New names do not change the reality of people's lives, for example, re–labelling the 'disabled' as 'differently abled' doesn't improve their material and social circumstances, and often new terms take on old meanings and connotations. Also, the poor and the disadvantaged have more serious and pressing things to worry about than "pedantic, linguistic niceties" (Molyneux, 1993, p 61). Finally, it is important to recognise that the way in which policies were implemented were often less than constructive, and easily ridiculed. In this respect, PC can be directly counterproductive and can strengthen reactionary ideas. Thus, attempts to combat abusive language can be important and significant, as they often represent an important shift from using, for example, the term 'coloured' to the term 'black' and from 'homosexual' to 'gay'. These developments represented great steps forward in terms of promoting pride and self-assertion among oppressed groups – and of course, were generated from within the oppressed community itself, so 'black was beautiful' and gays were 'out and proud'. However, there has to be a recognition that changing language will not necessarily alter the ideas or attitudes of others, and of course, an *imposed* linguistic code may have all the weaknesses but none of the strengths of self-identified language change.

The term PC, however, has been increasingly used by Right-wing politicians and sections of the media as a 'catch all' to ridicule and dismiss a whole set of values associated with equality and justice. Younge (2000b) offers an example of how it is used to openly express bigotry, when he cites comments of Judge Graham Boal, QC, at the Criminal Bar Association dinner in 1999 that an ideal candidate for the bar would have, "The breasts of a lesbian, the backside of a homosexual, and a large black penis". This was apparently a joke about PC, but on the back of the 'joke' stereotypes and oppression grow. Political correctness has become routinely stigmatised as an act of liberal dogma, described by Dennis O'Keefe in an Institute of Economic Affairs report as, "A mix of extremist egalitarian doctrines such as feminism, anti-racism and multiculturalism ... deeply threatening to social cohesion" (Younge, 2000b).

Although it is argued that the term is now used so widely that it is virtually meaningless, and that it is used to deride just about anything that the Right-wing do not agree with or do not like, PC nevertheless remains a very potent political weapon for those who wish to attack progressive changes in society. For example, in relation to social work developments, social workers were caricatured in the *Daily Mail* as:

> ... abusers of authority, hysterical and malignant callow youngsters who absorb moral-free marxoid and sociological theories to

undermine the family and encourage welfare dependency. (cited in Jones and Novak, 1999, p 155)

The attack on PC was never really primarily about the 'language issue' and the (sometimes ludicrous) excesses this produced. But ridiculing the supposed banning of 'black boards' or asking for a 'black coffee' was used as a stick to beat the wider and more general claims of anti-oppressive policies. So the nature of racism, discrimination, inequality and injustice were ignored, while it could be claimed that 'baa baa black sheep' (a nursery rhyme about peasants being forced to give their produce to their masters and the crown – the little boy down the lane) was being banned for not being PC. Whether this and other examples were ever true is in many ways less important than the fact that large numbers of people believed it could be true. The imposed policies and prescriptions of the PC reformists and managerialists had created a cover which their opponents could use to impose traditional and far more conservative forms of practice onto an increasingly demoralised profession.

As a result of these political attacks on anti-oppressive developments, institutional commitments to anti-oppressive practice within social work began to decline (Singh, 1996). This led to the revision of Paper 30 and the removal of its assertion of the endemic nature of racism in Britain. The fact that CCETSW succumbed to new-Right pressures to undermine the professional value base of social work, and failed to sustain anti-racist policies and practices, revealed its relative ineffectiveness as a state agency in offering independent direction. Webb stated that, "... CCETSW with its Chair and up to 25 members appointed by the Secretary of State is nothing, if not an extension of employer interests" (Webb, 1996, p 175).

In this political climate, anti-racism was further compromised. Political attacks on local authorities resulted in a decimation of the funding base of the black voluntary sector, and for black communities much of the goodwill built up in the 1980s was lost. Black people and voluntary groups grew increasingly cynical about the attitudes and approaches of local authorities, and there was the view that:

Local authorities ... have taken advantage of the political and ideological change during the Conservative era to effectively dump 'race' as an important issue. (Thompson, 1997, p 18)

As a result of these developments, anti-racist struggles were undermined and attempts were made to neutralise 'race' issues. It was not until the murder of Stephen Lawrence in 1993 that issues of 'race' and racism hit the political and public agenda again in a fundamental manner, and debates about institutional racism re-emerged. There was increasing evidence that the long struggles for change regarding anti-racist initiatives were failing to make any lasting impact, and criticism from black activists that 'race' issues were being pushed further down the agenda of social services departments (Singh, 1994). It gave rise to concern that the undermining of anti-racist developments would give social workers hostile to the changes the excuse they needed to ignore or avoid the issues.

However, the successful attack on CCETSW's initiatives, and the defensiveness, fear and insecurity among many social workers, also needs to be examined in relation to the "fragmentation, marketisation and residualisation of social services" (Canon, 1995, p 13) that has downplayed the helping, supportive, and continuing role of social work (Cheetham, 1992). Over the last decade social work has been overwhelmed by legislative change that has increased its regulatory and rationing role at the expense of its caring role. Social workers who intervene in the lives of the poor, disadvantaged and marginalised have increasingly had to meet diverse and dire human need in a climate of severe financial restraint – developments which have often resulted in a situation where demoralisation and exhaustion now characterise the social work profession (Jones and Novak, 1993).

The extent of the defeat of Paper 30 is also emphasised by the attempt to move social work education and training in the direction of being based on job-focused competencies, alongside a weakening and narrowing of the profession's education and research roots (Jones, 1996). As Canon states:

> person and social-based knowledge, experience and skills are being redefined in terms which reduce their value and which make social workers and their tasks more easy to manage in the workplace. (Canon, 1995, p 15)

Challenges to the intellectual and theoretical components of social work education and training were reflected in the comments of politicians such as Timothy Yeo, the then Junior Conservative Minister, who said in 1992 that, "social work education is far too preoccupied with 'ologies' and 'isms'" (cited in Jones and Novak, 1999, p 162). There has been increasing disquiet that these changes will involve the transmission of knowledge and skills for utilitarian objectives devoid of any critical reflection (Canon, 1995), making it even more onerous for students to implement anti-racist practice while on placement.

At the same time, the Conservatives were repeatedly questioning the usefulness of social work education and training. The academic component was increasingly under attack by the government, who favoured a move towards competency-based training, which undermined the role of social work education in promoting critical, analytical and reflective practice (Jones, 1994). This 'competence-based approach' to learning subordinates education to work, and reduces social work to 'measurable technical tasks'. The subsequent development of the National Certificate in Vocational Qualifications (NCVQ's) exacerbated this process by shifting power for determining professional standards from educational establishments to social work agencies (the very agencies which have been shown to be so inadequate in terms of implementing anti-racist practice).

Novak (1995) criticised these developments when he stated that:

> Doing anything betrays assumptions about the nature of the situation we are involved in, its causes and its solutions and what we have to do is make these assumptions explicit, to turn them into a theory and to test them against other theories ... it is also that practice can and should inform theory. Ideas that we develop about the world have always to be tested in the world if they are to be of any use, and if necessary subsequently modified in the light of that experience. (Novak, 1995, p 8)

However, a representative of CCETSW, in response to Novak (1995), defended the changes, when she commented:

> It would be entirely irresponsible for social work educators to train social workers for what we think they should be doing rather than for what they will actually have to do ... service users have to live in the real world of the market economy of welfare. Social workers are certainly not going to 'care' for them or 'respect' them more by burying their heads in the sand because we disapprove of the system ... we have to prepare competent practitioners who understand and can use and challenge the new systems to the best advantage of their clients while ensuring that their own practice is critical, reflective and firmly underpinned by social work values. (Weinstein, 1996, pp 34-8)

The subordination of theoretical awareness and professional qualifications was evident in CCETSW's decision in 1994 to abolish the requirement that practice teachers should be qualified social workers, and in the decision to remove probation training from the Diploma in Social Work.

Top-down policies

The PC impositions and CCETSW's anti-racist initiatives both reflect a similar political tradition: a reformist, gradualist politics of 'engineering social change'. The general goals of CCETSW's policies involved recognising the structural nature of oppression under capitalism, a position based on substantial sociological and theoretical evidence and knowledge. But the way the policy was imposed, like the PC imposed language codes, was never fully integrated into the work culture of social work agencies. Indeed, it was imposed in managerialist ways onto the profession. Paper 30 was a progressive policy initiative that was instigated and promoted by a small group of black and white professionals who were committed to the development of anti-racist social work practice, education and training. But CCETSW's policy always contained a major contradiction. CCETSW is a state agency, social work is a practice within which the dialectic of 'care and control' is crucial. Paper 30 denounced the endemic nature of racism in Britain and its institutional and structural nature, suggesting it was embedded in dominant social relations, and hence could not be removed until those social relations had been radically transformed. However, this is a revolutionary solution to the problem, and social work is not a revolutionary activity and, in part, many of its roles involve controlling and 'soft policing' (in probation work, for example) sections of the black community. The contradiction was in part revealed by Tony Hall who, in the face of the backlash, suggested the anti-racist initiative was merely a form of 'multiculturalism'. The policy was not built on solid foundations within the profession, linked in to other support networks. In the face of the backlash the initiative was abandoned with remarkable and undue haste. This change in direction met with little organised response from within the profession. The reason for this was that the policy was never 'owned' by social workers but imposed upon them, the commitment of the minority of radical social workers within the profession was not enough to defend it in the face of public, media, professional and government opposition.

EIGHT

Conclusion and recommendations

This book has focused on the development of CCETSW's anti-racist initiatives, as outlined in the *Rules and requirements for the Diploma in Social Work (Paper 30)* (1989). The aim has been to explore how CCETSW's anti-racist initiative came about, how it fared in practice, what reaction it generated, and what political response it produced. In doing so, it has been possible to offer an assessment of the successes and limitations inherent in 'progressive' top-down policy developments. This is important for, as Solomos and Back (1996) stated:

> ... there has been surprisingly little detailed analysis of the workings of public policy concerned with racial inequality and we still know relatively little about the workings of specific policies and programmes.... (Solomos and Back, 1996, p 76)

Paper 30 was a top-down policy initiative that attempted to deal with the manifestation of racism in social work agencies by imposing legitimate modes of practice onto social work students and practitioners. It did this by regulating training and assuming this would filter through to practice. One of the major concerns of the report has been to look at the successes and failures of this policy, and the barriers that prevented its constructive implementation and operationalisation. In doing so, it became evident that while anti-racist initiatives are clearly relevant to social work education and training in a society structured by inequality, policy initiatives by themselves do not necessarily invoke change in institutions such as social work agencies. It also became apparent that such policies are always vulnerable to counter-policies from political opponents hostile to anti-racist perspectives. By themselves then, top-down policy initiatives are relatively limited in the extent to which they alone can develop anti-racist practice within welfare agencies which themselves operate in ways that reflect and embody institutional racism.

An analysis of CCETSW's anti-racist initiative and the commitment to, and ability of, social workers to address racism and implement anti-racist social work practice also needs to be undertaken in the context of historical 'race-related' political developments. An analysis of such developments reveals that social work education, training and practice has tended to be dominated by individualistic and cultural theories of racism which do not focus on structural and institutional racism. Assimilationist, integrationist and multicultural perspectives that were favoured by governments from the 1960s to 1980s, had been unsuccessful in dealing constructively with racism in society and welfare institutions. These perspectives were influential in the development of equal opportunities policies that resulted in the employment of a few black professionals, but did not challenge structural and institutional discrimination (Gilroy, 1992). The pursuit of equal opportunities policies has also been characterised by a lack of clarity about what 'equal opportunities' means both ideologically and in practice.

Against this background 'anti-racism' developed within academic and social welfare discourse from the 1980s onwards. In Chapter Three I looked at why an anti-racist commitment should have been incorporated within social work education and training at a time when the 'Thatcher Project' was attempting to establish a new political hegemony within Britain. I suggested that the ideas and values of Thatcherism were always contested both within 'traditional' political locations (for example, Parliament and Local Government), and in the community at large (for example, via inner city riots, industrial disputes and community political initiatives). Part of this opposition was reflected in the growth of the 'reformist Left solution' in and around the Labour Party during the early 1980s, and the growth of women's and black sections which represented an acknowledgement of issues of gender and 'race' inequality by the Labour Party. As a result, issues of gender and racism became more visible in Labour Party discussions and documentation, and Labour controlled councils increasingly adopted equal opportunities policies. This resulted in a developing political culture within the Labour Party, local government and the equal opportunities community that stressed the racist nature of British society. This was one factor that helps to explain why, despite a political climate apparently hostile to 'progressive' politics, CCETSW could make a commitment to anti-racist social work education and training. From the 1980s onwards, authorities such as Hackney were also pressing CCETSW about the inadequacies of much professional training in preparing social work students for anti-racist work.

A second major element that influenced CCETSW's developments was the role played by black activists and academics in the welfare field. During the 1960s and 1970s a variety of black organisations were set up to organise against both discriminatory legislation and racist practices. Black groups were exposing the discriminatory practices that the black community faced at the hands of the British state, and were involved in resisting discriminatory and negative social welfare developments. Finally, the resistance to discriminatory welfare legislation also manifested itself in the social work arena, where black organisations and black practitioners had, over the years, been increasingly critical of the nature of social services provision for the black community that was characterised by negative and damaging stereotypes.

A third element was the development of various political and cultural organisations, which stressed black and white unity in grass roots politics to counter racism and the far-Right. The Anti-Nazi League and Rock Against Racism, for example, were significant in creating a youth culture within which anti-racism was positively promoted.

It was a combination of the wide anti-racist struggle, the input of black social workers, a growing awareness and critique of institutional racism within welfare agencies, and the rise of a counter-Thatcherite political opposition within the Labour Party, local government, and the equal opportunities community, which created the 'space' for CCETSW's anti-racist initiatives to develop. There had also been important staff changes in the upper management of CCETSW which were influential in increasing CCETSW's receptiveness to pressures from 'below' for anti-racist social work developments, for example, the appointment of Tony Hall as a Director, who had come from the British Association of Adoption and Fostering that had already developed anti-discriminatory policies around adoption and fostering.

As a result of such pressures, CCETSW demonstrated a serious commitment to look at routes to anti-racist social work practice, and began to question seriously why social work practice was so deficient in anti-racist initiatives. Subsequently, they formally adopted an anti-racist policy, developed Paper 30 which stipulated learning requirements in relation to anti-racist social work, and also produced Paper 26.3 which insisted that agencies and practice teachers should be able to facilitate anti-racist education and training. In 1988, CCETSW also launched its five year Curriculum Development Project (CDP), which it created in order to counter arguments from those hostile to anti-racist developments that there were no resources to facilitate anti-oppressive social work education and training. As a result, the CDP set itself the task of meeting these criticisms through the production of academic materials such as learning packs.

A key finding of the research was that racism was predominantly institutional in nature, and most social work professionals were unconsciously reproducing institutionally racist practices and procedures. There was evidence of differences among students and practice teachers in their commitment to anti-racism, and in their understanding of what it means at a conceptual and practice level. There were also differences in the ability and determination of students to confidently challenge racism. Nevertheless, all accounts demonstrated that, "without the active support of their agencies, individuals can only make a marginal impact on the quantity and quality of services provided" (Social Services Inspectorate, 1987, p 74).

There were three institutional barriers that acted as a deterrent to the implementation of anti-racist social work education and training: the under-representation of black clients, the under-representation of black staff, and the ineffectiveness of anti-discriminatory policies. Social work practice for the black community was built upon a series of negative stereotypical assumptions, and resulted in poor or inappropriate social work provision for black clients. It was assumed, for example, that Asian families were automatically able to provide adequate care, that Asian mothers were weak, or that mental ill-health was demonised in the Asian community, and the main barrier facing Asians looking for social work assistance was a linguistic one. Similarly, Afro-Caribbean mothers were thought strong and domineering and black youth aggressive. That such stereotypes could shape practice in a welfare institution is deeply worrying and suggestive of the extent to which a 'common-sense' racism is embedded within social work working culture. Black students interviewed were concerned that there was an assumption that they could work effectively with any black client regardless of gender, religion or other cultural differences, and that because they were black they were automatically 'race' specialists. The under-representation of black staff was compounded by their marginalisation within agencies. Section 11 workers in particular were treated differently (and badly), marginalised from the 'real' social work being undertaken within agencies. This had negative implications for black clients.

Finally, there was clear evidence of the inadequacy and ineffectiveness of anti-discriminatory policies in social work departments. If they existed, policies were usually no more than mere 'blueprints'. They had not been implemented. Resources had not been provided to ensure they were understood, activated and acted upon. There was no provision for education and training around the policy themes or their implementation. In essence, policies became part of a managerial strategy to 'pass the buck'; management had passed policy, they took the issues seriously, it was the workers who failed to implement it. Yet any such claims simply will not do. Workers and students rarely knew the policies (or even if they existed), and on the rare occasions workers or students attempted to implement them, senior management acted to undermine claims of racism and discrimination; those that raised the claims were depicted as troublemakers or having a 'chip on their shoulder'.

These institutional barriers affected how individuals coped with trying to implement CCETSW's anti-racist initiatives. Because of the failure of most social work agencies to deal with the manifestation of institutional racism, racist incidents were almost always undermined, denied or ignored. This led to a situation where challenging racism and/or dealing with it, became dependent on the personal and professional characteristics of individual students and practice teachers. There was a tendency for black and white students to react differently in this situation. Black students who had worked in white statutory agencies were much more aware of, and prepared for, the racism which they encountered on placement, and had often adopted strategies to deal with it. In contrast, less experienced black students tended to have more idealistic expectations regarding the anti-discriminatory nature of social work practice, especially in the context of the academic anti-discriminatory agenda, and the high profile which CCETSW's anti-racist initiative had at the time. Taking CCETSW's claims at face value produced anxiety and shock when faced with the reality of institutionalised racism within the agencies. Among white students, there was a general concern to implement anti-racist practice and apply theoretical considerations raised within the university. However, their ability to do so was mainly dependent on the attitude of their practice teacher. For example, even those personally and politically committed to anti-racist practice, found the racism that they witnessed in agencies very difficult or almost impossible to deal with if they had a hostile practice teacher. The students who were most alarmed regarding the racism that they witnessed in agencies were those with least experience, who tended to share the idealistic expectations of their inexperienced black colleagues. Other students who were keen to develop anti-racist practice while on placement were faced with a lack of information and awareness, which left them feeling confused, insecure, unsupported, and guilty when they failed to challenge racist incidents.

As discussed throughout this piece of work, the student's relationship with their practice teacher was a crucial factor in determining how 'safe' they felt in discussing anti-discriminatory issues. Practice teachers have the power to judge what is acceptable behaviour and practice, and have considerable influence in determining if anti-racist practice is part of the learning agenda. Practice teachers who participated in the research project were divided into three groups. First, there was a minority who were personally and professionally committed to and concerned about anti-discriminatory practice, and whose students were able to discuss issues of 'race' in a relatively secure environment. This group of practice teachers were 'open' to anti-racist developments and took black students' experiences of racism seriously. They were also willing to recognise gaps in their own knowledge, awareness and development. Many students considered such practice teachers to be 'radical', in contrast to a minority of more 'traditional' practice teachers who were overtly hostile to anti-racist practice, tended to deny or undermine the existence of racism in society, and saw no need for the development of anti-racist social work practice. However, the majority of practice teachers, although not hostile to anti-racism, nevertheless felt defensive, insecure and anxious about discussing issues associated with 'race' or dealing with racism. It would be wrong to conclude that these practice teachers were racist. Instead, they had been put in a position where they were expected to facilitate anti-racist learning experiences even though they lacked knowledge, awareness, education and training. As a result, although practice teachers were given almost exclusive power in assessing students' competency, they frequently reported feeling vulnerable and at times powerless during the placement process (Hackett and Marsland, 1997). For, as Cadman and Chakrabarti (1991) stated:

> Challenging values as deeply held as those which inform stereotypical assumptions and practices of agencies and workers alike is bound to generate resistance and hostility long before it awakens re-appraisal and changes in perception and behaviour. (Cadman and Chakrabarti, 1991, p 224)

Of course, all these issues have resource implications, resources for education, training and information provision, for example. Further, good practice teaching requires time and support, which many practice teachers found unable to provide in a climate of increased workloads, and when line managers were often unsympathetic to their role. If agencies view working with students as an additional burden to existing workloads (despite the fact that agencies get money for students and students do free work for them), then it is easy to see how the quality of placements has depended on the commitment of individual practice teachers.

Implications and recommendations

I finish by drawing together some of the implications of the research for future anti-racist strategies within welfare organisations. Although the research was based on social work training guidelines, it has wider significance.

Racism and social work

CCETSW's programme was a significant attempt to tackle institutional racism in one welfare organisation, the social work and social services departments of Britain's welfare state. Recent evidence highlights the continuing relevance of a need for such commitments, as Balloch (1997, p 45) found:

- 41% of black staff, social workers in particular, said they had experienced racism from service users or relatives;
- 27% of black staff said they had experienced racism from colleagues or managers;
- Most of those affected by racism had not received adequate help and support from their department.

Institutional racism involves addressing issues of black client and staff representation, ensuring that both are fully integrated into mainstream services and service provision, and not marginalised.

The CCETSW experience

CCETSW attempted to alter social work practice by changing the training programme and culture for social work students, and using practice teachers as a bridge to take these developments into the profession. Both these strategies were problematic. Students taught the 'theory' of anti-oppressive practice found themselves isolated, pressurised or confronted in a range of unexpected ways when they attempted to raise these issues on placement. Dominant work cultures and institutional norms were not altered by the students, but often adapted them to traditional modes of practice. Given that students had to pass the placement to attain the Diploma in Social Work, this is perhaps not at all surprising.

Practice teachers under CCETSW's Paper 26.3 were identified as central actors – key individuals expected to alter and facilitate the new practice. Yet practice teachers are drawn from social workers with a variety of values and conceptions of social work's role and functions. Some of these were in tune with CCETSW's innovations, most were intimidated by their own lack of experience and training, and some were overtly hostile. It is questionable whether the practice teacher (and the practice teacher/student relationship) was ever likely to be in a position to challenge significantly the work culture of agencies. However, if it was to succeed then, at the very least, any such strategy required a concrete engagement with practice teachers to address the concerns, build their confidence, create appropriate support networks, and rule out practice teachers who were inappropriate to the fulfilment of the new educational demands and training needs.

The 'isolation' of anti-discriminatory policies

CCETSW's initiatives were isolated from other developments and organisations outside social work looking to obtain similar goals. Welfare organisations exist in what can be termed a 'multi-organisational field' which include a range of welfare institutions, self-help organisations and community and political networks. Many of these institutions are grappling with anti-discriminatory issues. Shared knowledge and increased network support is a useful mechanism to overcome isolation within agencies.

The limitation of top-down policies

Finally, drawing each of the above points together is the method CCETSW adopted to implement change by imposing its strategy onto the profession 'from above'. Top-down policies, imposed in managerialist ways, in the context of resource cuts and increased workloads, often fail to engage with people's work and life experiences. There is no sense of 'ownership' among those at the workface and this leaves the policies vulnerable to counter-attack from political opponents. This is not to deny the importance of the policy initiatives, but to reveal the inherent weakness of this mode of imposition, and its complete failure to transform institutions and effectively challenge anti-racist practices and procedures. As Kwhali stated:

> It is ... quite unrealistic to expect social work institutions to be transformed into models of anti-discriminatory excellence simply

because new written requirements are placed upon them. (Kwhali, 1991, p 44)

That is, policies by themselves do not challenge institutional racism if they are decontextualised from social processes and do not connect with what is happening in the outside world. Instead, in order to be fully integrated into practice, anti-racist policies need to be more closely linked to wider counter-structural movements against racism, drawing on networks of support 'from below', from for example, black groups, trade unionists and other anti-racist activists, to generate a feeling of ownership through education and engagement with all social workers or other welfare workers (and not simply those on any 'liaison committee'). Such developments have resource implications, but if there is a serious commitment to tackling institutional racism, resources should be provided. Further, this is of necessity an ongoing commitment because as Gambe et al (1992) noted:

Anti-racism should not be seen as offering certainties, absolute for all time. We have to be ready to change and adopt our ideas in the light of experience, debate and developments. (Gambe et al, 1992, p 10)

Bibliography

Ahmad, B. (1988) 'The development of social work practice and policies on race', *Community Care*, 14 January.

Ahmad, B. (1989) 'Self-definition and black solidarity', *Social Work Today*, 11 May.

Ahmad, B. (1990) *Black perspectives in social work*, London: Venture Press.

Ahmad, I.U. and Atkin, K. (1996) *'Race' and community care*, Buckingham: Open University Press.

Ahmed, S. (1991) 'Developing anti-racist social work education practice', in Northern Curriculum Development Project (ed) *Setting the context for change*, London: CCETSW.

Alibhai-Brown, Y. (1993) 'Social workers need race training and not hysteria', *The Independent*, 11 August.

Anderson, J. and Cochrane, A. (eds) (1989) *A state of crisis: The changing face of British politics*, London: Hodder and Stoughton.

Arnold, E. and James, M. (1988) 'Finding families for black children in care: a case study', *The Jewish Journal of Sociology*, vol 30, no 2, December.

Association of Directors of Social Services/CRE (1978) *Multi-racial Britain: The social services response*, London: ADSS/CRE.

Balen, R., Brown, K. and Taylor, C. (1993) 'It seems so much is expected of us – practice teachers, the Diploma in Social Work and anti-discriminatory practice', *Social Work Education*, vol 12, no 3.

Ballard, R. (1979) 'Ethnic minorities and the social services', in V.S. Khan (ed) *Minority families in Britain*, London: Macmillan.

Balloch, S. (1997) *The social services workforce in transition*, London: National Institute of Social Work.

Barclay Report (1982) *Social workers, their roles and tasks*, London: Bedford Square Press.

Barker, M. (1981) *The new racism: Conservatives and the ideology of the tribe*, London: Junction Books.

Barker, M. and Beezer, A. (1983) 'The language of racism – an examination of Lord Scarman's report on the Brixton riots', *International Socialism*, vol 2, no 18, Winter.

Bebbington, A. and Miles, J. (1989) 'The background of children who enter local authority care', *British Journal of Social Work*, vol 19, no 5.

Benhabib, S. (1995) 'From identity politics to social feminism', in D. Trend (ed) *Radical democracy: Identity, citizenship and the state*, New York, NY: Routledge.

Ben-Tovim, G., Gabriel, J., Law, I. and Stredder, K. (1986) *The local politics of race*, Basingstoke: Macmillan.

Benyon, J. and Solomos, J. (eds) (1987) *The roots of urban unrest*, Oxford: Pergamon Press.

Bhaduri, R. and Hughes, R. (1987) *Race and culture in social services delivery (a study of 3 social services departments in the north west)*, London: Social Services Inspectorate.

Bhat, A., Carr-Hill, R. and Ohri, S. (1988) *Britain's black population (a new perspective)*, Hants: Gower.

Blackburn Borough Council (1996) *The changing face of Blackburn and Darwen*, Blackburn: Blackburn Borough Council, Economic Development Unit.

Blackburn, R. (1997) *The making of new world slavery*, London: Verso.

Boddy, M. and Fudge, C. (1984) *Local socialism? Labour councils and new left alternatives*, London: Macmillan.

Bowling, B. (1999) 'Facing the ugly facts', *The Guardian*, 17 February.

Bradford Commission (1996) *The report of an inquiry into the wider implications of public disorders in Bradford which occurred in Bradford on 9, 10 and 11 June, 1995*, London: The Stationery Office.

Bradford Post Qualifying Partnership (1991) 'Antiracism requirements and the Diploma in Social Work', in CCETSW (ed) *One step towards racial justice (the teaching of anti-racist social work in Diploma in Social Work programmes)*, London: CCETSW.

Bridges, L. (1994) 'Tory education: exclusion and the black child', *Race and Class*, vol 35, no 1.

Brodie, I. (1993) 'Teaching from practice in social work education: a study of the content of supervision sessions', *Social Work Education*, vol 13, no 2.

Brown, C. (1984) *Black and white Britain: The third PSI survey*, London: Heinemann.

Brown, C. (1992) 'Same difference: the persistence of racial disadvantage in the British employment market', in P. Brahm, A. Rattansi and P. Skellington (eds) *Racism and anti-racism: Inequalities, opportunities and policies*, London: Sage Publications.

Bruegel, I. and Kean, H. (1995) 'The moment of municipal feminism: gender and class in 1980s local government', *Critical Social Policy*, vol 44/45, Autumn.

Bryan, B., Dadzie, S. and Scafe, S. (1985) *The heart of the race*, London: Virago.

Butler, B. and Elliott, D. (1985) *Teaching and learning for practice*, Aldershot: Gower.

Cadman, M. and Chakrabarti, M. (1991) 'Social work in a multi-racial society: a survey of practice in two Scottish local authorities', in CCETSW (ed) *One step towards racial justice (the teaching of anti-racist social work in Diploma in Social Work programmes)*, London: CCETSW.

Callinicos, A. (1985) 'The politics of "Marxism Today"', *International Socialism*, vol 29.

Callinicos, A. (1987) *Making history*, Cambridge: Polity Press.

Callinicos, A. (1989) *Against post-modernism*, Cambridge: Polity Press.

Callinicos, A. (1993) *Race and class*, London: Bookmarks.

Callinicos, A. (1995) *Theories and narratives*, Cambridge: Polity Press.

Callinicos, A. and Simons, M. (1985) *The miners strike of 1984/5 and its lessons*, London: Socialist Worker.

Cambridge, A.X. and Feuchtwang, S. (eds) (1990) *Anti-racist strategies*, Aldershot: Avebury.

Canon, C. (1995) 'Enterprise culture, professional socialisation and social work education in Britain', *Critical Social Policy*, vol 42, Winter.

Castles, S. and Miller, M.J. (1993) *The age of migration*, London: Macmillan.

CCETSW (Central Council for Education and Training in Social Work) (1989a) *Rules and regulations for the Diploma in Social Work (Paper 30)*, London: CCETSW.

CCETSW (1989b) *Regulations and guidelines for the approval of agencies and accreditation and training of practice teachers (Paper 26.3)*, London: CCETSW.

CCETSW (ed) (1991a) *One step towards racial justice (the teaching of anti-racist social work in Diploma in Social Work programmes)*, London: CCETSW.

CCETSW (1991b) *Rules and requirements for the Diploma in Social Work (Paper 30)* (2nd edn), London: CCETSW.

CCCS (Centre for Contemporary and Cultural Studies) (1982) *The empire strikes back: Race and racism in 1970s Britain*, London: Hutchinson.

Cheetham, J. (1987) 'Racism in practice', *Social Work Today*, 27 September.

Cheetham, J. (1992) 'Social work and community care in the 1990s: pitfalls and potential', in R. Page and J. Baldock (eds) *Social Policy Review 5*, University of Kent, Social Policy Association.

Clarke, J. (1980) 'Social-democratic delinquents and Fabian families – a background to the 1969 Children and Young Persons Act', in National Deviancy Conference (ed) *Permissiveness and Control*, London: Macmillan.

Clarke, J. (ed) (1993) *A crisis in care (challenges to social work)*, London: Sage Publications.

Cohen, S. (1996) 'Anti-Semitism, immigration controls and the welfare state', in D. Taylor (ed) *Critical Social Policy: A reader*, London: Sage Publications.

Cook, D. (1998) 'Racism, immigration policy and welfare policing: the case of the Asylum and Immigration Act', in M. Lavalette, L. Penketh and C. Jones (eds) *Anti-racism and social welfare*, Aldershot: Ashgate.

Coombe, V. and Little, A. (1986) *Race and social work (a guide to training)*, London: Tavistock

Cox, P. and Hirst, G. (1995) 'Placements as a site of oppression: some evidence and evaluation', *Social Work Education*, vol 14, no 1.

CRE (Commission for Racial Equality) (1989) *Racial equality in social services departments: A survey of equal opportunities policies*, London: CRE.

Curtis, L. (1984) *Nothing but the same old story (the roots of anti-Irish racism*, London: Information on Ireland.

Davidson, W. (1999) 'The trouble with ethnicity', *International Journal of Social Work*, vol 84, Autumn.

Daye, S.J. (1994) *Middle class blacks in Britain*, London: Macmillan.

de Gale, H. (1991) 'Black students' views of existing CQSW and CSS schemes: 2', in Northern Curriculum Development Project (ed) *Setting the context for change*, London: CCETSW.

de Souza, P. (1991) 'A review of the experiences of black students in social work training', in CCETSW (ed) *One step towards racial justice (the teaching of anti-racist social work in Diploma in Social Work programmes)*, London: CCETSW.

Dempsey, M. and Divine, D. (1991) 'Learning from experience', in CCETSW (ed) *One step towards racial justice (the teaching of anti-racist social work in Diploma in Social Work programmes)*, London: CCETSW.

Denney, D. (1983) 'Some dominant perspectives in the literature relating to multi-racial social work', *British Journal of Social Work*, vol 13, no 2.

Denney, D. (1991) 'Anti-racism, probation training and the criminal justice system', in CCETSW (ed) *One step towards racial justice (the teaching of anti-racist social work in Diploma in Social Work programmes)*, London: CCETSW.

Dominelli, L. (1988) *Anti-racist social work*, London: Macmillan.

Donzelot, J. (1979) *The policing of families*, London: Hutchinson.

Draper, H. (1966/97) *The two souls of socialism*, London: Bookmarks.

Duncan, D. (1986) 'Eliminate the negative', *Community Care*, 5 June.

Ely, P. and Denney, D. (1987) *Social work in a multi-racial society*, Aldershot: Gower.

Ferguson, I. and Lavalette, M. (1999) 'Social work, postmodernism, and Marxism', *European Journal of Social Work*, vol 2, no 1.

Fox-Piven, F. and Cloward, R.A. (1977) *Poor peoples movements – Why they succeed and how they fail*, London: Pantheon.

Francis, E. (1991) 'Mental health, anti-racism and social work training', in CCETSW (ed) *One step towards racial justice (the teaching of anti-racist social work in Diploma in Social Work programmes)*, London: CCETSW.

Fryer, P. (1984) *Staying power: The history of black people in Britain*, London: Pluto.

Fryer, P. (1988) *Black people in the British empire*, London: Pluto.

Gambe, D., Gomes, J., Kapur, V., Ranger, M., Shubbs, P. and Dutt, R. (1993) 'Improving practice with children and families: a training manual', *Children and Society*, vol 9, no 3.

Gamble, A. (1988) *The free economy and the strong state*, London: Macmillan.

Gilroy, P. (1987) *There ain't no black in the union jack*, London: Hutchinson.

Gilroy, P. (1992) 'The end of anti-racism', in J. Donald and A. Rattansi (eds) *Race, culture and difference*, London: Sage Publications.

Ginsburg, N. (1992) *Social divisions of welfare*, London: Sage Publications.

Gitlin, T. (1994) 'The rise of identity politics', in N. Mills (ed) *Legacy of dissent*, New York, NY: Simon and Schuster.

Gordon, P. (1992) 'Black people in the criminal law (rhetoric and reality)', in P. Braham, A. Rattansi and R. Skellington (eds) *Racism and anti-racism*, London: Sage Publications.

Gore, C. (1998) 'Inequality, ethnicity and educational achievement', in M. Lavalette, L. Penketh and C. Jones (eds) *Anti-racism and social welfare*, Aldershot: Ashgate.

Gramsci, A. (1971) *Selections from prison notebooks*, London: Lawrence and Wishart.

Guardian, The (2000) 'Race: a special report one year after MacPherson', 2 February, p 21.

Hackett, S. and Marsland, P. (1997) 'Perceptions of power: an exploration of the dynamics in the student–tutor–practice teacher relationship within child protection placements', *Social Work Education*, vol 16, no 2.

Hall, S. (1980) 'Race, articulation and societies structured in dominance', in UNESCO (ed) *Sociological theories: Race and colonialism*, London: UNESCO.

Hall, S. (1985) 'Realignment or what?', *Marxism Today*, vol 29, no 1.

Hall, S. and Jacques, M. (1983) *The politics of Thatcherism*, London: Lawrence and Wishart.

Hall, S., Critcher, C., Jefferson, T., Clarke, J. and Roberts, B. (1978) *Policing the crisis: Mugging, the state and law and order*, London: Macmillan.

Hardwick, N. (2000) 'Piling on the hysteria', *The Guardian*, 11 February.

Harman, C. (1999) *A people's history of the world*, London: Bookmarks.

Harris, V. (1991) 'Valves of social work in the context of British society in conflict with anti-racism', in Northern Curriculum Development Project (eds) *Setting the context for change*, Leeds: CCETSW.

Hasan, R. (2000) 'Riots and urban unrest in Britain in the 1980s and 1990s', in M. Lavalette and G. Mooney (eds) *Class struggle and social welfare*, London: Routledge.

Heinemann, B.W. (1972) *The politics of the powerless*, London: Open University Press.

HMSO (1991) *Women in social work*, London: HMSO.

HMSO (1994) *Social Trends 24*, London: HMSO.

Hobsbawm, E. (1977) *The age of capital 1848-1875*, London: Sphere.

Holborow, M. (1999) *The politics of English*, London: Sage Publications.

Husband, C. (1980) 'Culture, context and practice: racism in social work', in R. Bailey and M. Brake (eds) *Radical social work*, London: Edward Arnold.

Husband, C. (1991) '"Race", conflictual politics, and anti-racist social work: lessons from the past for action in the 1990s', in Northern Curriculum Development Project (ed) *Setting the context for change*, London: CCETSW.

Hussan, R. (2000) 'Riots and unrest in Britain in the 1980s and 1990s: a critique of dominant explanation', in M. Lavalette and G. Mooney (eds) *Class struggle and social welfare*, London: Routledge.

Institute of Race Relations (1980) *Equal opportunities: A report by the ILEA inspectorate*, London: ILEA.

Jenkins, G. (forthcoming) 'Competing strategies in the anti-nazi struggle', in C. Barker, A. Johnson and M. Lavalette (eds) *Constructing strategies, transforming identities*, Liverpool: Liverpool University Press.

Jessop, B., Bonnett, K., Bramely, S. and Ling, T. (1988) *Thatcherism*, Oxford: Polity Press.

Johnson, A. (2000) 'The making of a poor people's movement: a study of the political leadership of Poplarism 1919-1925', in M. Lavalette and G. Mooney (eds) *Class struggle and social welfare*, London: Routledge.

Johnson, N. (1990) *Reconstructing the welfare state*, Hertfordshire: Harvester Wheatsheaf.

Joint Council for the Welfare of Immigrants (1995) *Immigration and nationality handbook*, London: JCWS.

Jones, C. (1983) *State social work and the working class*, London: Macmillan.

Jones, C. (1993) 'Distortion and demonisation: the right and anti-racist social work education', in *Social Work Education*, vol 12, no 30.

Jones, C. (1994) *Dangerous times for British social work education*, Paper delivered at the Congress of the International Association of Schools of Social Work, Amsterdam.

Jones, C. (1996) 'Anti-intellectualism and the peculiarities of British social work', in N. Parton (ed) *Social work and social theory*, London: Routledge.

Jones, C. (1998) 'Setting the context: Race, class and social violence', in M. Lavalette, L. Penketh and C. Jones (eds) *Anti-racism and social welfare*, Aldershot: Ashgate.

Jones, C. and Novak, T. (1993) 'Social work today', *British Journal of Social Work*, vol 23.

Jones, C. and Novak, T. (1999) *Poverty and the disciplinary state*, London: Routledge.

Joyce, P., Corrigan, P. and Hayes, M. (1988) *Striking out: Trade unionism in social work*, London: Macmillan.

Kwhali, J. (1991) 'Assessment checklists for DipSW external assessors', in CCETSW (ed) *One step towards racial justice (the teaching of anti-racist social work in Diploma in Social Work programmes)*, London: CCETSW.

Lancashire County Council Planning Department (1986) 'Lancashire's Asian community', *Monitor no 38*, Lancashire: Lancashire County Council.

Langan, M. (1993) 'The rise and fall of social work', in J. Clarke (ed) *A crisis in care (challenges to social work)*, London: Sage Publications.

Lavalette, M. (1997) 'Marx and the marxist critique of welfare', in M. Lavalette and A. Pratt, *Social policy: A conceptual and theoretical introduction*, London: Sage Publications.

Lavalette, M. (1999) 'The "new sociology of childhood": child labour, childhood, children's rights and "children's voice", in M. Lavalette (ed) *A thing of the past? Child labour in Britain in the nineteenth and twentieth centuries*, Liverpool: Liverpool University Press.

Lavalette, M. and Mooney, G. (1990) 'Undermining the "north–south divide?": fighting the poll tax in Scotland, England and Wales', *Critical Social Policy*, vol 29, Autumn.

Lavalette, M. and Mooney, G. (1999) 'New labour, new moralism: the welfare politics and ideology of New Labour under Blair', *International Socialism*, vol 85, Autumn.

Lavalette, M. and Mooney, G. (2000) *Class struggle and social welfare*, London: Routledge.

Lavalette, M. and Pratt, A. (1997) *Social policy: A conceptual and theoretical introduction*, London: Sage Publications.

Lavalette, M., Penketh, L. and Jones, C. (1998) *Anti-racism and social welfare*, Aldershot: Ashgate.

Law, I. (1998) 'Sharpening the conceptual tools: racial and ethnic inequalities in housing and policy', in M. Lavalette, C. Penketh and C. Jones (eds) *Anti-racism and social welfare*, Aldershot: Ashgate.

Lewankin, R.C., Rose, S. and Kamin, L.J. (1984) *Not in our genes: Biology, idealogy and human nature*, New York, NY: Pantheon Press.

Lister, M. (1997) *The European union and the south*, London: Routledge.

Ludlam, S. and Smith, M.J. (eds) (1996) *Contemporary British conservatism*, Basingstoke: Macmillan.

MacDonald, I., Bhavni, T., Khan, L. and John, G. (1989) *Murder in the playground: The report of the MacDonald inquiry into racism and racial violence in Manchester schools, (The Burnage Report)*, London: Longsight Press.

MacPherson, W. (1999) *The Stephen Lawrence Inquiry Report*, Cmnd 4262, London: HMSO.

Malik, K. (1996) *The meaning of race*, London: Macmillan.

Manning, P. (1990) *Slavery and African life*, Cambridge: Polity Press.

Mansfield, M. (2000) 'White on black', *The Guardian*, 17 February.

Manthorpe, J. and Stanley, N. (1997) 'Private placements in social work education: Opportunity or oppression', *Social Work Education*, vol 6, no 1.

Marfleet, P. (1999) 'Nationalism and internationalism in the new Europe', *International Socialism*, vol 84, Autumn.

McCrudden, C., Smith, D.J. and Brown, C. (1991) *Racial justice at work*, London: Policy Studies Institute.

Miles, R. (1982) *Racism and migrant labour*, London: RKP.

Miles, R. (1989) *Racism*, London: RKP.

Miles, R. (1993) *Racism after race relations*, London: Routledge.

Miles, R. and Phizacklea, A. (eds) (1979) *Racism and political action in Britain*, London: RKP.

Miles, R. and Phizacklea, A. (1984) *White man's country*, London: Pluto.

Modood, T. (1988) 'Black, racial equality and Asian identity', *New Community*, vol 14, no 3.

Molyneux, J. (1993) 'The politically correct controversy', *International Socialism*, vol 61, Winter.

Mooney, G. (1998) 'Remoralizing the poor? Gender, class and philanthropy in Victorian Britain', in G. Lewis (ed) *Forming nation, framing welfare*, London: Routledge.

Mullard, C. (1991) 'Towards a model of anti-racist social work', in CCETSW (ed) *One step towards racial justice (the teaching of anti-racist social work in Diploma in Social Work programmes)*, London: CCETSW.

NACRO (National Association for the Care and Resettlement of Offenders) (1993) *Awaiting trial – The final report*, London: NACRO.

Norton-Taylor, R. (1999) *The colour of justice*, London: Oberon Books.

Novak, T. (1995) *Ideas in action. Thinking about a real social work curriculum*, vol 14, no 4.

Oppenheim, C. (1993) *Poverty: The facts* (2nd edn), London: Child Poverty Action Group.

Owusu-Bempah, J. (1989) 'The new institutional racism', *Community Care*, 14 September.

Patel, N. (1991) 'The curriculum development project: model and process 1988-1990', in Northern Curriculum Development Project (ed) *Setting the context for change*, London: CCETSW.

Penketh, L. (1998) 'Anti-racist policies and practices: the case of CCETSW's paper 30', in M. Lavalette, L. Penketh and C. Jones (eds) *Anti-racism and social welfare*, Aldershot: Ashgate.

Penketh, L. and Ali, A. (1997) 'Racism and social welfare', in M. Lavalette and A. Pratt (eds) *Social policy: A conceptual and theoretical introduction*, London: Sage Publications.

Pinker, R. (1999) 'Social work and adoption: a case of mistaken identities', in T. Philpot (ed) *Political correctness and social work*, London: Institute of Economic Affairs.

Ramdin, R. (1987) *The making of the black working class in Britain*, Aldershot: Gower.

Refugee Council (1997) *'Just existence': A report on the lives of asylum seekers who have lost entitlement to benefits in the United Kingdom*, London: Refugee Council.

Rex, J. (1973) *Race, colonialism and the city*, London: RKP.

Rex, J. and Moore, R. (1967) *Race, community and conflict*, Oxford: Oxford University Press and Institute of Race Relations.

Rex, J. and Tomlinson, S. (1979) *Colonial immigration in a British city*, London: RKP.

Roys, P. (1988) 'Social services', in A. Bhat, R. Carr-Hill and S. Ohri (eds) *Britain's black population*, Hants: Gower.

Runnymede Trust and the Radical Statistics Race Group (1980) *Britain's black population*, London: Heinemann.

Saggar, S. (1992) *Race and politics in Britain*, Hertfordshire: Simon and Schuster.

Scarman, Lord (1982) *The Scarman report: The Brixton disorders*, Harmondsworth: Penguin.

Seebohm Report (1968) *Report of the committee on local authority and allied personal social services*, Cmnd 3703, London: HMSO.

Singh, G. (1994) 'Anti-racist social work: Political correctness or political action', *Social Word Education*, vol 13, no 1.

Singh, G. (1996) 'Promoting anti-racist and black perspectives in social work education, practice and teaching', *Social Work Education*, vol 15, no 2.

Sivanandan, A. (1981) 'From resistance to rebellion: Asian and Afro-Carribean struggles in Britain', *Race and Class*, vol 23, no 2-3.

Sivanandan, A. (1982) 'Waiting for Scarman', *Race and Class*, vol 23, no 4, Spring.

Sivanandan, A. (1985) 'RAT and the degradation of black struggle', *Race and Class*, vol 26, no 4.

Sivanandan, A. (1990) *Communities of resistance*, London: Verso.

Sivanandan, A. (1991) 'Black struggles against racism' in Northern Curriculum Development Project (ed) *Setting the context for change*, London: CCETSW.

Sivanandan, A. (1998) Commentary 'The making of home to the beat of a different drum', vol 39, no 3, Jan-March.

Skellington, R. and Morris, P. (1992) *'Race' in Britain today*, London: Sage Publications.

Smith, C. and White, S. (1997) 'Parton, Howe and post-modernity: A critical comment on mistaken identity', *The British Journal of Social work*, vol 27, no 2, April.

Smith, S. (1994) 'Mistaken identity or can identity politics liberate the oppressed', *International Socialism*, vol 62, Spring.

Social Services Inspectorate (1987) *Report of the conference on race and culture in personal social services*, London: DHSS.

Solomos, J. (1991) *Black youth, racism and the state*, Cambridge: Cambridge University Press.

Solomos, J. and Back, L. (1996) *Racism and society*, Basingstoke: Macmillan.

Steadman-Jones, G. (1971) *Outcast London*, Oxford: Oxford University Press.

Stokes, I. (1996) 'Black practice teachers: a review of some literature and its meaning for social work education and practice', *Social Work Education*, vol 15, no 2.

Strang, S. (1995) 'Paperwork' Inside (Black Overrepresentation), *Community Care*, 23 February, 1 March.

Thompson, A. (1997) 'Black power', *Community Care*, 24 July/30 July.

Thompson, N. (1993) *Anti-discriminatory practice*, London: Macmillan.

Troyna, B. (1992) 'Can you see the join? An historical analysis of multicultural and anti-racist education policies', in D. Gill, B. Mayor and M. Blair (eds) *Racism and education – Structures and strategies*, London: Sage Publications.

Troyna, B. and Hatcher, R. (1992) 'Racist incidents in schools: a framework for analysis', in D. Gill, B. Mayor and M. Blair (eds) *Racism and education – Structures and strategies*, London: Sage Publications.

Wadsworth, M. (1998) *Comrade sak (Shapurji Saklatvala MP, a political biography)*, Leeds: Peepal Tree Press Ltd.

Walton, C. (1975) *Women and social work*, London: RKP.

Webb, A. (1980) 'The personal social services', in N. Bosanquet and P. Townsend (eds) *Labour and equality: A fabian study of labour in power 1974-79*, London: Heinemann.

Webb, D. (1996) 'The state, CCETSW and the academy', in N. Parton (eds) *Social theory, social change and social work*, London: Routledge.

Weinstein, J. (1996) 'A reply to Tony Novak', *Social Work Education*, vol 15, no 1.

Williams, B. (1996) 'Probation training: the defence of professionalism', *Social Work Education*, vol 15, no 3.

Williams, J. (1985) 'Redefining institutional racism', *Ethnic and Racial Studies*, vol 8, no 3.

Wilson, E. (1992) *A very British miracle*, London: Pluto.

Wilson, M. (1989) 'Equal service for a multi-racial community', *Social Work Today*, 6 July.

Woodward, K. (1997) *Identities and difference*, London: Sage Publications.

Woodward, W. (2000) '£5,000 bond to stop Asian "illegal settlers"', *The Guardian*, 31 January.

Wrench, J. and Solomos, J. (1993) *Racism and migration in Western Europe*, Oxford: Berg Publishers Ltd.

Younge, G. (2000a) 'A year of reckoning', in *The Guardian*, 'Race: a special report one year after MacPherson', 2 February, p 21.

Younge, G. (2000b) 'The badness of words', *The Guardian*, 14 February.